My fight against Ebola in the Republic of Guinea

Dr. Sakoba KEÏTA

My fight against Ebola in the Republic of Guinea

L'Harmattan

L'Harmattan, 2022

5-7, rue de l'École-Polytechnique - 75005 Paris

www.editions-harmattan.fr

ISBN : 978-2-14-031629-6
EAN : 9782140316296

The purpose of this book

I am writing this book in this post-ebola period for several reasons, the first of which is out of a duty to bear witness to my compatriots and secondly, in response to numerous requests from national and international partners. I give here all my experiences learned from the management of epidemics. I have managed more than 35 in the country, including Ebola, which aroused the emotion of everyone and brought about a flawless mobilization of the Guinean population. Being one of the leaders in this response, I feel indebted to write this book-testimony, to reflect on this epidemic, its management and the challenges faced; to take stock of the solutions provided, the lessons learned, and our actions related to our response to various epidemics.

This writing, I produce as a testimony, as I have mentionned. I am also doing it for the new generation, that has the right to know what really happened in Guinea between 2014 and 2016, so that it can learn lessons for the future. Because, if some countries in Africa have experienced several epidemics, such as the Congo which was in its tenth epidemic in recent years, one might believe that other events will occur in Guinea after Ebola and COVID-19, even if I do not wish for them. The possibilities exist and the best thing, at least I think so, is to prepare for those eventualities, instead of waiting for misfortune to knock on our door again before reacting. We must prepare, because only preparation can prevent the onset of an epidemic or reduce its effects if it does occur.

This is the deep desire that prompted me to submit to the writing of this testimonial book. It is for our children that I am writing it. It is for young people that I am writing it, so that they can one day become managers of future events, because these are realities that we do not often learn in our schools, in which teaching is very classical. It is case studies that help to discover certain field realities in order to adopt future strategies.

I could have written this book a long time ago. Which brings us back to the question of: "why now?" In fact, three years ago, I wanted to write this book, but my daily activities in the fight against various diseases did not give me the time for it. My first strategy was to find collaborators to help me, because writing is not an easy exercise. This is the place, for me, to make it clear that I am not a writer in the truest sense of the word. As there was a change in the management of the epidemics, I had more free time, which allowed me to take the plunge. After dealing with Ebola, I was able to delegate some of my responsibilities to trustworthy people who still report to me today, every morning. Before, I was in charge of data management, treatment, and logistics among other things. Today, I'm more of a manager than a direct executor. This is what allowed me to have time to devote myself to writing this testimony, which I consider a duty.

I expect critical comments on this book from my readers. Above all, I expect the new generation to take ownership of the content of this book to be the next soldiers against the diseases that will take our country by storm. I expect better management of the next epidemics that will occur in Guinea.

I expect from them the same patriotism and the same commitment to future fights against diseases that threaten our collective life and our national sovereignty.

I expect to see thousands of young Guineans and Africans do better than Sakoba in the epidemic response after learning from my journey. Because, if I am writing this book, it is to warn young people, to prepare them on all fronts to prevent our country from the next health crises. I am comforted today to know that the number of people publishing testimonials is increasing.

In this book, I report on the services rendered to the nation, on what I have done in the Ebola response, with my whole team, of course. I am very satisfied to have fulfilled this duty. Everyone has their limits, and this testimony is interested in the budding heroes who, I hope, will do even better than me in the fight against epidemics in the Republic of Guinea, and why not in any country of Africa and the world?

Since my childhood, I have dreams for my country. Some have come true, and others are in progress. For my country, I have always prayed to God to give me the means to serve to the satisfaction of the Guinean population, thus making my contribution in the construction of our country. Since I started working in the health system in 1981, I have taken a lot of actions, but it was Ebola that pulled me out of the shadows. My dream for Guinea is for its people to always be in good health and to benefit from a very efficient health system with health workers who respect the deontology and ethics of the medical profession. I wish we could develop our structures to have fewer infectious diseases, less chronic diseases such as leprosy and tuberculosis, and less malaria, in short, to have healthy citizens who will devote themselves to work to raise our country to a harmonious and respectable level of development. Finally, I dream of seeing Guinea appear among the emerging countries and, why not, among the most developed countries in the world. I wish all possible happiness to the Guinean population, starting with good health. This is why I often go to medical schools to help train future doctors who will take over.

Presentation of Dr Sakoba KÉÏTA

I am Dr. Sakoba Keïta, Director General of the National Health Security Agency (ANSS) and I was born on June 8, 1954 in N'Zerekore, a town located in southern Guinea. My father's name was Bakary Keïta and my mother's Tiranké Kaba. In 1960, I entered the "Mamadou Konaté" elementary school in N'Zérékoré. Then, in 1965, I continued my secondary studies in the capital, Conakry, more precisely in the commune of Kaloum at the school of the center which was then close to the Senegalese mosque. There, I lived with my uncle, the late Mamoudou Keïta, who was a driver at the Ministry of Planning. He drove the minister Alioune Dramé during the first regime of Ahmed Sékou Touré. My uncle, my father's younger brother, had agreed with my father to send one of my mother's children to study with him in Conakry.

My father was a trader and worked with white traders during the colonial era. He sold palm nuts.

My schooling at the French school was encouraged by my mother, who was from a family versed in religious beliefs and wanted her sons to be educated. Being her first son, I was therefore schooled and at the same time, I went to the Koranic school where I learned to read the Koran. My father lived in Sanankoro, in the sub-prefecture of Babila, prefecture of Kouroussa. One day, he was designated by his father to honor the payment of the capitation tax for his whole family. It is in this context that he undertook trips from prefecture to prefecture in this palm nut business in order to earn the money necessary to pay the family tax.

In N'Zérékoré, my father benefited from the kindness of the late Elhadj Mory Sangaré, who welcomed him and offered him a part of his concession. There is a very old saying in Guinea, that the latter said to him: *"As long as you live, I will guarantee the friendship with you because of the feeling that binds us and you will be able to stay here as long as you remain on this land".* This is how this piece of land was built by my father. The first children of my father were born in this concession, in the district of "Kouté Aplou".

My mother is originally from Kankan, more precisely from the sub-prefecture of Karifamoria. As for her ancestors, they lived six kilometers from Kouroussa (Meningui) and three or even four generations of their lineage settled there, but it must be remembered that they are originally from Kankan. My mother lived with her paternal uncle, who was a civil servant during the colonial era and who was a government employee. It was my maternal grandfather who provided for her education. And it was during one of my father's stays in Kankan that he met the woman who would later become my mother. The bond between them grew little by little between them.

In elementary school, I was a pretty good student. I still remember some teachers who marked me during my school career. Among them was a European woman who taught at the elementary school "Mamadou Konaté". At each exam, she gave a small gift to the laureates and, as a result, each one of us invested much more in our studies. That is how she pushed us to be interested in mathematics.

In high school, I was also influenced by my math teacher, Mr. Fofana, who is no longer with us. My perception of life, as well as my behavior, were influenced by one of my philosophy teachers, Mr. Ismael Condé, who taught at the high school “2 Octobre”. He continues, even today, to give advice to young people to instill moral values. What impressed me the most about this teacher was his honesty, his integrity and especially his way of analyzing things. He often has very solid and convincing arguments. His morality allowed him to hold high positions under the first regime in Guinea.

In my education, my uncle imposed strict rules on me. He regretted his illiterate state. He demanded that I study every night, especially reading. He would go to my school to check on my behavior and would not hesitate to whip me if I was not in the top five in my class. Almost every day he would talk to me about his regret for not going to school and encourage me to study to save our family's honor. He made sure to apply this rule to all his children.

My uncle's house was just like my real parents' house because his wives provided me with all the necessary care. We spent our vacations in the interior of the country with my parents, where I received the warmth of my mother. In those days, during vacations, the state provided the schools with a lot of money, and our parents did not have to pay for our transportation or a large part of our schooling. Even school supplies were given to the students. We also benefited from free health care.

During vacations, in my village, a certain tradition applied. The students came to the village to share the life of the villagers, the communities. As for me, I spent three months in Sanankoro and took part in the work in the fields and in the fonio harvest. Sometimes, we even went behind the oxen in the bush. These vacations allowed me to keep a certain love for my village, my cousins, and my parents. I am still very attached to this village that I loved at the time when we danced "Doundoumba" and when we went to the river to bathe. These are some of the memories I have of my village, which I continue to visit. Whenever I have a little time, I meet my cousins there, who have grown older, like me, but our complicity has remained intact. I don't regret these harmonious moments that allowed me to build my personality. Today, I still remain attached to my land while contributing to its development.

I spent only one year at the school of the center in Kaloum and, when I obtained my certificate of primary studies, I went to spend my last cycle of college, as well as high school, at “2 Octobre”. Thus I spent almost seven years in this establishment. In high school, where I chose geochemistry, I passed my baccalaureate with honors and in 1973 I received a scholarship to Cuba where I did my university studies. I wanted to teach mathematics because of my preference for exact sciences, and my ease in mathematics, physics, and chemistry since primary school, but life decided otherwise.

In 1968, when I was only 14 years old, I had a serious accident during a soccer game. An opponent in the middle of the game hit my face with his knee, the shock was so strong that it caused my whole head to swell up. My vision remained blurred for a long time. I was treated by the late Dr. Hadjatou Sylla with whom I spent three or four years of care. When I came for my care, I sometimes spent two to three hours waiting, which gave me time to observe the doctors in the exercise of their profession. I was immediately attracted to this profession. It should be noted that the injuries caused by the accident changed my life forever because they were irreversible. It was a great disappointment for me. Fortunately, I had a friend who gave me a book entitled *"The Support of the Subconscious Mind in the Life of a Man"*. This book allowed me to forget about my illness and to go on with my life as if it had never happened. I finally convinced myself that I could achieve all my goals. After the accident, my father wanted me to stop studying so that intensive reading wouldn't damage my eyes any further. But my uncle and mom were very keen for me to finish my studies. Eventually, I gained courage, redoubled my efforts, and reduced my distractions so that I could devote more time to reading. For three years, this incident changed me and made me doubt of my future.

This ordeal convinced me that I could become a great person for my country. So, I decided to study medicine to better understand my health issues and see how to avoid making my handicap worse. During the three years of high school, I regrouped and continued with the same momentum. I was always in the top five in my class. When the results of the baccalaureate were announced, I was confident in my success, but did not know to what extent. In the end, with honors and finishing in the top ten of the Republic, I was exempted from having to compete be qualified for university.

At first, we wer supposed to continue our studies in Algeria. Finally, Cuba was retained. We were forced to change country, because the class of Guinean students who had preceded us, had run away, never returning to Guinea as planned. We were very happy with this decision because Cuba was a foreign and distant country. I had never traveled before and was excited to see a country outside of Africa.

Before undertaking this journey, I went to visit my mother. My family was no longer living in N'Zerekore. She had moved to Kouroussa, where my father wanted to live after the death of his older brother in 1972. In the large family, the right of descent is applied. When the oldest brother dies, the brother who succeeds him takes the "throne of wisdom". It was my father's turn to be the patriarch of his family, hence his choice to be closer to his family. At first, he settled in Kankan before moving to Kouroussa.

I knew Kouroussa well, having gone there regularly on vacation since I was 12 years old. Around 1966, I would spend at least 3 months there, every year. With my friends, I did folk dances, went to the creek, hunted, and cultivated. These moments are dear to me and made me love this part of Upper Guinea. We listened to the tales of the village as well as many proverbs on the love of the homeland, solidarity, and virtue. One of our proverbs really shaped me and, in a way, materialized my wish to join an enterprise after my retirement: It is the story of a man who caught a fish with which he developed a very solid friendship. When he caught it, he put it in a well. The fish made a lot of babies, so it could not continue to live in the well. He asked his master to open roads that lead to the river. His master agreed and on the way to the river, in thanks, the fish offered some of his babies as food. The man refused, saying that their friendship meant too much to him and that he preferred the fish kept his young with him. He could not eat the flesh of his friend's young. The fish continued to sing and procreate. It is because of this story that I started a fish farming project in my village.

But this is not the only reason. In 2016, with the advent of Ebola, I did a kind of touristic trip with the support of the head of state, Professor Alpha Condé. I went to France where I spent two weeks, to Canada, to the United States, and in some African countries. In the United States, I was asked what was the thing that was most important to me and what I would I like to do to help my community. I had just finished a book on a demographic health survey, which showed that malnutrition in our country was close to 50%. Moreover, I remembered not being able to eat freshwater fish when I had gone to my village during a Tabaski celebration for a whole week, despite insisting. I could not find any fish to buy in my village or in the surrounding area even if the biggest river of the country, the Niger River, runs through our region.

So, I told the Americans that I would like to do some farming. I needed their expertise to know, between poultry or fish, which were more resistant to diseases. They recommended fish. I was able to visit a fish farm in Atlanta, which I found very appealing. That day, I listened and recorded everything I saw, and advice I received.

After the visit, I considered replicating a similar center in Guinea, in collaboration with the fish farming center I visited. Today, even if I have not yet begun to market my fish, I have a fish farm that could, I think, produce enough fish in the near future to help the women of my village to increase their income through sales and thus fight against malnutrition by providing the necessary proteins for the development of children. I also plan to promote community fish farming at the level of the prefecture and even the whole country. All these factors have allowed me to build my idea to set up this small fish farming center.

My years of study in Cuba went very well. At the time, there was a lot of media hype and political slogans. We read tomes of the late President Sekou Touré, which instilled in us a great patriotism. When we arrived in Cuba, we felt the same enthusiasm for Fidel Castro, who was a great speaker. He was able to motivate his audience with his speeches. Our behavior was influenced by this. We dedicated a month of our vacations to field work, what they called voluntary work. I participated in the clearing of sugar cane fields. This contributed greatly to the shaping of our personality. We took a sociology course entitled: "Man and his environment", in other words, how man must adapt to his environment. This course helped us in a way to facilitate our adaptation and has helped my adaptation to any environment.

At the time, Cubans were not demanding of Guinean students materialistically. We were given money which allowed us to buy a few things and also to go out and recreate every Saturday. From a health point of view, every six months, everyone had a systematic examination. This allowed me to detect illnesses in time and treat them. For example, I was able to get ten of my teeth filled, which lasted for more than twenty years. This is how most of the foreign students did not experience any serious illness in Cuba.

We were really integrated with the Cubans because in each group of students there was at least one of us, which helped us to learn the language and to understand the habits and customs of our hosts.

Several delegations from Guinea came to visit us in Cuba, among which the Minister of Education at the time, Mamady Keita, who was my father's cousin visited us two or three times and encouraged us. Back then, without phones, we could only receive news from our country by radio broadcasts, available only after midnight because of the time difference. Mamady Keita liked to say that youth is the future of a country. He gave us a lot of patriotic love, that became part of us and that most of us used to serve our country upon return.

Personally, I think Fidel Castro was a great man, he seduced me for the love he had for his country. When I listen to some of his speeches today, I still find them relevant to the balance of power that exists in this world where the richest continue to abuse the naivety of the weakest. Fidel fought for a certain social balance. He has always supported the less fortunate and the weakest. This attitude of refusing luxury and share the life of the weakest by blending into society appealed to me. I shared the work in the fields with his older brother Raül. This period marked me a lot. I also followed his story "sierra maestra", in the mountains where he began his fight for the liberation of his country and where he was warmly welcomed by the population. All of these stories caught our attention and contributed to our personal development so that we could, despite all the knowledge that we acquired, remember that we came from a village and that it is our duty to use our knowledge for the welfare of our people.

His example influenced the behavior of many of my friends when they returned to Guinea. Many had opportunities to go into exile but refused to do so and stayed to participate in the construction of our country. As for me, I received my doctorate in general medicine in Cuba, in August 1980.

The first choc came at our return, when after finishing the agropastoral farm campaign (FAPA) where everyone had to do a short internship, we were forbidden to serve in Conakry or the surrounding cities. This was a real shock for me because I wanted to work at the Ignace Deen Hospital in Conakry, in the pneumology department with Professor Oumou Younoussa Sow, with whom I had been in contact. Unfortunately, at that time, to respond to the shortage of doctors in the interior of the country, all fifty of us were sent to reinforce the prefectures of the interior.

Seyfoulaye Diallo, one of our fathers of independence, was then Minister of Health. He was very demanding and insisted that his criteria be respected. Finally, we accepted his decision considering that he was doing it to help the interior of the country by sending useful competences. A month later, we were all in our assigned post.

My father was the older brother of Minister Mamady Keita but the effects of the influence of relationships for exams and assignments were not too visible. When I left for Cuba, he did not know me. When I graduated with honor, as I had the name of his father, he wanted to know me. Someone explained to him that I was the son of his brother, and he offered me a few suits when I left for Cuba. So, when I returned, he was very happy with me and gave me his business card to help me have my wish granted to stay in Conakry. We were four or five people who had similar recommendations, but as I said earlier, our dear father Sayfoulaye Diallo, who was very demanding, began by spreading to the interior the people with recommendations. As soon as my name was pronounced, he sent me to Siguiri. The one who came right after me went to Lola. And so on. Those not recommended already knew their fate. When others saw that the most highly recommended were sent fair away in the interior, they started to hide their letters of recommendation! I wish that this kind of decision would continue in the hearts of our future leaders and even of those of today so that there would be less favoritism, in the transfer as well as in the management of human resources of our country. This created a feeling of equity, a feeling of being managed together. Unfortunately, the evolution of times and mentalities have led Guineans to abandon the good habits that our leaders had then.

So here I am serving in Siguiri, my first post, where I never had any difficulties, socially or workwise, even if the working conditions were difficult. I had never been to Siguiri before, but I adjusted quickly to the district. Imagine a person who studied in Havana, transferred to a region where he is asked to work without electricity. Even in the hospital, we had to operate with flashlights. I had never been confronted with such practices during my apprenticeship in Cuba. Honestly, we did not think it was possible to work in such conditions. However, watching my Guinean colleagues excel in this environment, perform medical procedures and save lives, we had no choice but to follow suit. Notwithstanding these material difficulties, I quickly adapted to the life there and to the working conditions that were offered to me. Our technical knowledge greatly contributed to the success of such an enterprise, not to mention my reading of *"Man and his environment"*.

I got married in 1984. In 1981, I was 27 years old and as any young person, fun and distraction prevailed with many songs, patriotic slogans, solidarity and work requirement. I have to admit that our elders provided a good frame of reference by teaching us to love our country, to give ourselves for our country by doing a lot of voluntary work. It was a time of good security. When night fell, no one attacked anyone else. There was a lot of solidarity between people and less greed because when we did missions in the villages, the villagers took care of us by putting us up and feeding us. There was no such thing as a per diem, and we did not ask for it because we did not even know it existed. Life was so filled with solidarity. And we felt better in such an atmosphere.

I only stayed 11 months in Siguiri, from January to November 1981. I was promoted. After three months spent at the hospital of Siguiri in internal medicine, there was a need for doctors for prevention, and the regional director of Health of Siguiri sent me to work with endemic diseases. This was a new shock for me, having completed by internship in internal medicine and having to deal with diseases I had not not studied, especially since there was no leprosy in Cuba. I had to comply, as no one at that time could question the decision of his boss. I adapted by attending a workshop on prevention, management, and vaccination problems, etc.

Sleeping sickness which is known as trypanosomiasis in Guinea is caused by a parasite called the African trypanosome, is still present in Guinea, even if reduced by deforestation and new methods of fighting against this disease. But, back then, trypanosomiasis was very common in Guinea. When this disease infects a person, he sleeps a lot. Even when he washes himself for example, he falls asleep. If the disease is not treated quickly, it can take very severe forms and even lead to death.

Young and enthusiastic, I answered a lot of questions and was quickly noticed by the ministry's officials. They named me as chief doctor of prevention at the level of the General Commissariat of the Revolution (C.G.R) of Kankan in charge of practically all of Upper Guinea. I thus obtained my first service vehicle. I returned to Kankan where I spent almost 14 years in this new position. Then the region was divided into two administrative regions, Kankan and Faranah. After the split, I was only responsible for the five districts of Kankan.

In 1994, when the new region of Mamou was created, I was promoted to regional health inspector of Mamou, where I stayed from 1994 to 1997. In 1997, I was then assigned in the same capacity to the Boké region, where I stayed for three years. In 1998, I went to Benin, to complete a master's degree in public health at the Regional Institute of Public Health in Cotonou. Upon return in 2000, I was promoted to the position of national coordinator of the leprosy control program. I had rubbed shoulders with this disease in Siguiri. I had dedicated 22 years of my professional life to the fight against leprosy. This expertise in leprosy proved to be crucial in helping me coordinate the Ebola crisis and in my future management. I joined this position at a very difficult time in a climate of mistrust and mismanagement. An Indian working at the WHO had these words that have stayed with me forever: "to improve your management and the management of people, you have to know how to use the carrot and stick ". By "carrot", he meant that you must know how to thank and reward those who work well. The "stick" is there to punish but you must never lower it, it must remain in the air. Even today, I still admit that I sometimes raise my voice, but I always hesitate to go as far as sanctioning.

I started the fight against leprosy in 1981. All the positions I held between 1981 and 2000 gave me the opportunity to conduct many studies. I even specialized at the Marchoux Institute in Bamako, now the National Center for Support in the Fight against the Disease (CNAM), where I did a three-month internship in leprology in the 1990s. If I can speak of a health program that has contributed to the construction of my personality, it is the leprosy program, through which I developed a relationship with the "Raoul Follereau" foundation. In the field of fight against leprosy, we had three grand foreign partners : the "Raoul Follereau" foundation, which was in charge of Lower Guinea and Upper Guinea, the Philafrican mission in Forest Guinea, basede in Macenta, and the Order of Malta in Middle Guinea. Being responsible for the Upper Guinea area, I benefited from a lot of training from Raoul Follereau and have read his books. I found him to be very patriotic. He taught us that if you want to be happy, all you have to do is make others happy. He asked the French government to just give him the equivalent of the price of a bomber to end leprosy in the world.

Before, lepers were sent outside the villages, and in some countries, they were even confined in enclosures, without any care. They died of starvation and other epidemic diseases. It is during his visits to these leprosy sites, even if he was not a medical doctor then, that he noticed these deplorable living conditions. This awareness led him to dedicate the rest of his life to this debilidating disease.

In Guinea, too, most leprosy clinics were located on the outskirts of towns. He began to mobilize enough resources through his connections to fund studies to find drugs for leprosy. Today, thanks to him, we have drugs that can shorten the time to cure leprosy to 6 months or even 1 year. The impact of leprosy in Guinea has been greatly reduced from more than 60,000 leprosy cases to less than 500 cases detected today. This is the work of the thinker Raoul Follereau whom I regret not having been able to know personally. On the other hand, I met his spiritual son, André Récipon, whose son, Michel Récipon, was president of the French Association Raoul Follereau. I was able to meet him during his visits to Guinea.

This is how, not wanting to work on leprosy at the beginning of my medical studies, I develoed love and compassion for lepers and dedicating myself to it. In Cuba, when told to study exotic diseases, I argued that I wanted to work in internal medicine. I did not agree to extend my stay by one month to study infectious diseases. But fate made me dedicate 22 years of my medical service to leprosy. Thanks to Follereau's writings and my regular contact with leprosy patients, I cared for them. I wondered if I were in their place, how I would behave. This disease must absolutely disappear from the world. I know many Guineans who have been handicapped by this disease and who have not been able to continue their life project. I am very proud to have been able to participate in this fight and to have helped to break down some of the taboos surrounding leprosy.

In Upper Guinea, people said that when a leprosy stain was seen on a person's skin, his or her marriage was in jeopardy, and since leprosy had no cure, the person was condemned to be handicapped for the rest of his or her life and thus unable to support a family. We succeeded in breaking this taboo by taking the guarantee that the patient could be cured. We did not know the origin of most diseases because micro-organisms live in nature. We only know today that we can prevent leprosy because there are countries which have succeeded in completely eradicating this disease. There are institutions such as the Sasakawa Foundation, which is committed to the complete elimination of leprosy in the world. It is one of the first financial partners in the fight against leprosy, and together with many other humanitarian associations, it continues the fight against this disease that who has handicapped and continues to ostracize many human beings on the planet. This bacterial disease is very pernicious and demands an urgent fight. Before, there was no cure, but nowadays, with new molecules, thansfully, we can cure them. There are also other drugs to fight against diseases of the same family as leprosy such as microbacteria, tuberculosis ... which all have negative effects in this world, but that researchers and doctors are investing themselves in controlling.

I like to read and listen to the radio, especially the health programs on Radio France Internationale (RFI) and (RTL). When you hold certain positions of responsibility, you must keep a general knowledge of your field. In the positions I have held, I have always been involved in the fight against epidemics and always in the front line.

At the time, the most frequent epidemics in Upper Guinea were menigitis and measles. As early as 1981, I contributed to the fight against these diseases. Then, we also had a few episodes of cholera, again in Upper Guinea. When I arrived in Mamou and Conakry, I also had to deal with yellow fever. Recently, I had to deal with Lassa fever, then Ebola and now we are dealing with the COVID-19 pandemic with our national teams and international support. Must I mention there were also a few epidemics of H1N1 influenza in 2009 and 2010? I was very busy.

Since I benefited from certain positions of responsibility, especially after my departure from Kankan, I had little opportunity for leisure except on special occasions or meetings. My pilgrimage to Mecca also kept me away from distractions. I miss those rare moments; man must take time to relax. Today, I watch television. There were very hard times especially during Ebola, but also at the start of the COVID-19 crisis when my work pace was very fast. I would leave my house at 5am and stay at work until about 8pm. With the traffic jams to get out of the city of Conakry to the suburbs, I would only get home at 10 pm. I was exhausted and it took its toll on my family.

But, I always continued to be concerned about being available to people. When you are in a position of responsibility, you must think about how to communicate, how to master all the facets of the disease in order to reassure people on a factual basis and rely on logical reasoning. My daily effort consists of finding a balance in order not to frighten people without trivializing the disease too much either. Emotional decisions must be avoided.

When I was regional health inspector in Mamou, we organized a national meeting on the review of the Expanded Program on Immunization, Primary Health Care and

Essential Medicines (EPI-PEVSS). I made many presentations. This attracted the attention of the organizers who came from Conakry and in particular of the Minister of Health at the time, the late Dr. Kandioura Dramé. When he saw my presentation of the financial evaluation of my health center, which had a very low deficit rate compared to the money we had set aside for the reserve fund. He appreciated my rigorous management, and it was at that moment that the Minister took an interest in me. He allowed me to benefit from a scholarship for a master's degree in public health at the INSP of Cotonou. Upon my return, he promoted me to coordinator of the leprosy program at that time. That is how I came to Conakry in 2000 to exercise this position for 8 years.

After many years of experience in public health, enriched by numerous trainings I was given the position of head of the prevention division. In this position, I managed nearly 30 epidemics in collaboration with the program (PEVSSPME). I was also in charge of surveillance, i.e., the collection of health data and alerts. It is in this context that Ebola found me. I provided information on the disease and wrote daily bulletins on the evolution of the epidemic. We conducted a lot of meetings at WHO where I was always on the front line.

In September 2014, the government decided to set up an Ebola coordination. Given my role, I was selected to be the coordinator of the response to this disease.

Then, epidemics were followed by a national health crisis committee managed and presided by Professor Sidiki Diakité. I was then in charge of the secretariat, of surveillance, and of data collection of this committee. During our meetings, I provided information about the situation and sometimes, with partners, we proposed intervention strategies.

At the end of my studies, when I returned from Cuba, like most students, I came back with many books. I came back to my village with three suitcases of books and very few suits.

The villagers, seeing my suitcases, thought that I had come back with a lot of gifts for them. So, I was well received. People came to greet me and friends from the village were curious to see what my suitcases could contain. When I opened them, I had very few visitors! They forgot that it was through these books that I could strengthen my personality and get everything I wanted. I even had to give the Cuban outfit I was wearing to one of my relatives. By telling you this episode of my life, I want you to understand that in fact, I came back to my country without money, with only a suit and books. It took me four years to prepare for my wedding while I saved up the necessary money. My elder brother, the late Moussa Keita, came to my aid to build my wedding suitcase. It is only in 1984, that I could finally get married. Today, I am the happy father of four children, the youngest of my children was born in 1998. I have three daughters and one son who have all finished their studies and have even started working. In terms of education, I thank my wife who was able to devote part of her time to the education of our children. My wife's name is Bintou Diakité. She studied agriculture at the University of Kankan, which is where I met her in 1981. In 1984, after the army took over, she registered to become a teacher. Later, she started to teach in Kankan and then she was transferred first to Mamou. From there, she moved to Boké. Today, she continues to teach at the communal education office in Ratoma.

Thanks to God, all my children were able to study. With my daily occupations, I did not have time to teach them, we only met a few times as a family to keep the family link. Today, two of my children work in France, but I always told them not to forget where they come from, nor their duty to continue to contribute to the development of their country.

At each gathering, I tell them my story where I started at the bottom of the ladder with my uncle who was a driver and did not have enough money to help me. The value of our society is the love for the country more than for material gains. I also encourage them to earn money by the sweat of their brow and not easily, to invest in productive work and not in the bad business that many young people do today by ripping people off. I am also against illegal immigration and the fact that young people consider the West to be heaven on earth. I had the opportunity to visit the West several times and I could see the dark side that many people ignore. There are miserable people there, people who have no shelter and who sleep under bridges. Some of them go out to pick apples and do cleaning when these are the same jobs they refused to do back home. Generally, what they earn from these activities does not allow them to invest in other activities and those who have remained in Guinea live better than they do. This is the case of some Guinean soccer players who fail there because the proportion of people succeeding in this field is very insignificant to be cited as an example. Personally, I think that we should not dream to this extent. In the mining areas of Upper Guinea, many young people lose their lives for a few grams of gold, while there are other sectors of activity more promising.

A griot says "that there are three periods which characterize the process of acquiring wealth, namely:

1. **Obtain money**: this period requires efforst, perseverance, and sometimes risks for your life or integrity.
2. **Keep the money**: a difficult period because you have the rists of theft, fraud, depreciation, or fire tht are frequent in Africa where many keep their money at home.
3. **Invest:** This period requires judicious choices, objectives, a mechanism of guaranteed management, perhaps an insurance.

The poor conception or management of this last period can bring you to desolation and see all your efforts poorly rewarded, and forbide you to receive profit from your gains.

That said, at each step of our fight to live better, the search for financial resources must be guided by a project with clear and pertinent objectives. One must take into account the advice of experimented people and put in place some mechanism of guarantee or insurance. These measures are necessary and indispensable for the realization of youth dreams. We do not recommend hurrying and seeking easy methods of enrichment that often finish with deceptions, adventures like migration, and even conflict with the law. All these steps require training and patience.

I think that we can take an example from some people who have been able to create farms and who are fulfilling themselves in field work. It is true that their earnings are often small, but they manage to provide for their needs. We have a duty to educate these young people who see life as a mirror where everything is easily won, when in reality nothing is easily acquired. I was only discovered in Guinea after more than 30 years of good and loyal service to the Nation and yet it was Ebola that put my personality in the spotlight. Before this disease, I had fought against many other diseases. I had been on the radio several times, but it had never attracted the attention of people. So, I ask the youth to be aware and to be inspired by those who succeeded in their country. Young people should have very clear goals in life by looking for role models who have succeeded in their country.

I read a book that presenting the 5 keys to success: love for our country and love for our loved ones. All religions say that we should share a small percentage of our wealth with our parents. One of the keys to success is perseverance, paying the price to get what we want in life. It is very difficult to succeed without accepting this sacrifice of pain and endurance. For example, the man who invented the lamp failed 9999 times and every time he was told to give up, he replied that he never failed, but rather discovered ways not to make a lamp. He made his lamp for on his 10,000th attempt. This means that it takes perseverance to achieve your goals, but it also takes a leader or a reference.

Personally, I have references in the Ministry of Health, where there are people I admired for their integrity and their behavior. These people helped build my personality. Professor Mahy Barry helped me a lot with trainings and wise advice. The late Professor Mohamed Salif Sylla, who was the Secretary General of the Ministry of Health, helped me construct myself. Professor Pathé Diallo was my thesis director. Mrs. Sow, born Oumou Younoussa Bah, for almost 20 years, not only participated in my training but also helped me a lot. I want to also mention the late doctor Captain Seny Diakite who supported me a lot. Also, the Malian doctor Sekou Amadou Diallo came from time to time to Guinea to supervise us and participated in our training. I would not like to omit Dr. Prof. Daumerie who was my trainer at the Marchoux Institute in Bamako and who also supervised us. He trained us in the fight against leprosy. Late Professor Gatef (Institut de Pharo, Marseille), a Frenchman, also contributed to my training. All these people instilled in me cardinal values and helped build the Sakoba of today.

When I look back and learn from the past and think of the author of the *five keys to success*. I thank my parents who taught me the values of courage and perseverance. I realize that my parents' blessing has led me to success. This is a great satisfaction for me. At the end of the Ebola disease, I was allowed to express myself and I understood that without this responsibility, I would not have been able to express this hidden talent that I had in me. I thank Professor Alpha Conde for giving me this opportunity. The President of the Republic trusted me. Other partners have supported me during difficult moments when I could have lost courage. This is the place to thank them fully for their solidarity with me. But beside that,

I feel a sense of sadness, I keep a taste of unfinished business, I know I could have done better.

I would like to correct this regret if time and energy allow. We need to improve our health care system and even though I am on the verge of retirement, I would like to see a health care system with more humanism, with less greedy doctors. I think we will build a system that will meet the primary needs of these doctors so that they are more concerned about the health of the sick. I am sure that God will inspire me to find a solution one of these days. Unfortunately, it is a virus that continues to spread in my country.

I must admit that my stay in Cuba and my wife, were determining factors. Although I had to respect certain African customs, I managed to get along with her to the point of helping her as soon as I could with housework. I established a climate of collaboration to solve our problems. I put her in confidence and as she is Diakhanké (Marabout) and comes from a family of scholars, finally, a great complicity was established between us and allowed us to accept each other. I was able to entrust her with the management of our household when I was taking care of the outside world and the family needs. She is a great support to me and during my periods of discouragement, it is she who supports me morally as well as my dear mom. When I have difficulties, I confide in them because most of the time, as I am impulsive and quickly get discouraged, they know how to find the right words to make me see reason. My wife gives me advice and most of the time, I end up regaining courage and understanding that I should not make decisions out of anger.

My mom is still alive and is 87 years old. I hardly grew up with her. I only spent 11 years with her, but I have always kept in touch. Not only did she give birth to me, but she is also my main advisor and I call her frequently because she needs to hear from me for reassurance. In my Mandingo culture, I was taught that to succeed in life, you had to take care of your parents. Unfortunately, I I did not have the opportunity to take care of my father who died in 1987, except for the one time he was very sick. I had just started working when he died, so I was not able to give back to him as I do now for my mom. Today I can take care of her, I was able to take her to Mecca and whenever she is sick or has a health problem, all her children and I do what is necessary to help her through this difficult time.

I have 4 children, my first daughter was born in 1987, the same year my father died. She is a social worker and currently lives in France and works in a hospital. She is married to one of our compatriots and has 2 children. She left Guinea after the first year of university. She has remained attached to her country and her children have come to visit us twice. My recommendation is that I would not want her to stay in France for good and that I would like my offspring to contribute to the development of Guinea and not by staying away but by being present in the country.

My second daughter was born in 1989 in Kankan. She is the mother of 3 children and also lives in France. Currently, she is preparing with her husband to return to Guinea through small projects in collaboration with companies. As for my third daughter, she was born in 1993 in Kankan and lives with me in Guinea. She works at the Ministry of Health. My fourth child, a boy, was born in 1998. He studied economics in Morocco. He has finished his master's degree in economics in France and is preparing to return to Guinea in 2021, God willing.

My attachment to my homeland is explained by historical facts told by griots praising our ancestors like Soundiata Keita. I am a descendant of his younger brother Mandé Mory. We were taught to be warriors, to fight for our country. I was very much seduced by our predecessors like the history of

Sékou Touré and Sayfoulaye Diallo who joined hands with little culture because most of them had not gone to university. When they expressed themselves in French, we realized that their level exceeded that of us academics today. They agreed to regain their freedom. I have read about slavery that humiliated our people and many of them became aware of the wrongs of colonial domination and have dedicated themselves body and soul to the liberation of our societies. I have always found that these people deserved to be accompanied in their struggle. It is true that political independence has been achieved but the economic independence that should consolidate this policy is not yet achieved. Therefore, I think that we (as a new generation) must continue what our predecessors started by making sure that there is patriotic love and by making sure that we can give the little we have for the development of our country, like many other emerging countries where intellectuals have joined hands and have boosted their internal development, making the glory of their people today. I am referring to China, India, Brazil, etc. And why not Guinea, Senegal, or the Ivory Coast?

I greatly admire developed countries and I would also like my country to be one. It is this vision that I have of Guinea and this love for my country that led me to give up many positions of responsibility that were offered to me abroad. For example, in 2002, I was chosen by a company as an expert to go and serve abroad. I was very excited by the financial offer that was made to me at the time, but when I asked my wife and mother for advice, they immediately dissuaded me and reminded me that the children needed me for their education. At that time, because of the scarcity of telephones, my mother, fearing that she would not hear from me again and that she would die without seeing me, did not give me her approval. It is for these reasons, among others, that I gave up my expatriation.

I think that our society would benefit from modifying certain customs in order to be more humanitarian and to diminish a little this character which encourages us in the obscurantism. I sometimes make interventions on this subject towards the karamokos and the sages. I would like to see a world that is much more transparent and honest in its relationships. We must work to find appropriate solutions to our problems of development and living together. We must banish jealousy among us and as my uncle used to say: "God loves everyone". Everyone has a destiny, what you could not win, your son could perhaps get it, you never know. This is for example my case, I obtained what my parents could not obtain, and I learned a proverb in Mamou which says this: "every family gives birth to three types of children": the "young brother", his "equal" and his "big brother". As far as the education of children is concerned, one must always be the equal or the older brother of one's father, but when one is the younger brother of one's father, it would mean that the inheritance left by the latter has been poorly maintained, sometimes even sold, or is the reason for a conflict in court. I ask the new generation to think about this proverb. I therefore beg the new generation to think carefully about this proverb. They must not destroy the heritage that our elders have left, I mean patriotic love, community, love of neighbor, etc. Selfishness is not part of the African heritage. We are united by birth, we must build our people, where each one brings his contribution. Being equal to your father is to preserve the inheritance that has been bequeathed to you, but to preserve it, it is necessary to know it. Hence the need to be in the company of the elders, to read the books they have left. We must move away from ethnocentrism and easy gain in the exercise of our professions. There are Guineans who falsify diplomas to have access to the civil service or to services whereas in our time, we denounced people who copied in class.

We must cultivate integrity that was the hallmark of our parents' behavior. We must do everything to keep the right reflexes. As for the father's big brother, he is the one who will not only reinforce these values but also inculcate others such as new technologies in the respect of our values while improving our living conditions. I pray to God that the new generation will follow in this direction because each of us must leave a mark like the most respected of our predecessors. They were able to get us out of slavery and it is regrettable to see today that many do not know what slavery is to the point of regretting even our independence.

No people in the world like to be slaves because no one would like to belong to a master who has the right of life and death over them.

This is what I wish for my community in order to raise the nation higher because Guinea deserves that its values be preserved. We must water the tree that our predecessors planted so that it bears good fruit for the people of Guinea. I said to myself that we should not be too pessimistic, I know that during youth, there are also these moments of dream and among them, there are some who distinguish themselves by their patriotic love, by their investment for the development of Guinea. They are many among the women and among the leaders. I think that the youth will take the right path and it is up to us to identify the shortcomings, but the cement is integrity. The ability to accept each other and to refuse to reject the other.

Even though I am Malinke, I speak perfect Sousou and Malinke. As for Guerze, I have lost some of it over time. My wife speaks Sousou, Malinké, Diakhanké and Poular. I would like to praise the love of solidarity and I would like the heritage left by our elders to be maintained. At the time, to better cement our traditional ties, people from different regions married each other. Young people must integrate these values. There is a saying that you should never fight against your uncle's family. If your parents come from two different regions, you will never take up arms against the families of your two parents. Let's not get carried away by the greed of some of our leaders who want to do their dirty work at any cost. This is the message that I wanted to convey to all Guineans to make Guinea a real country where it is good to live for all its children. We must love one another. Merit must be above a sense of belonging.

I know very well that our predecessors were true warriors because they fought and succeeded in overcoming these difficulties of identity. We can do it too.

The history of Ebola

In 2014, Ebola was reported for the first time by the Regional Health Directorate of N'zérékoré, following the death of the director of the hospital in Macenta. His funeral was the subject of much mobilization of friends, relatives. During this first investigation, we noted many deaths and saw that the disease came from Miliandou, in Guéckédou, where the cousin of the deceased fell ill while providing care to some people in the village. This investigation revealed that the disease started in December 2013.

The real cause of the disease could not be established. We only knew that it was a disease with a high mortality rate.

When I received this worrying information, as chief of surveillance, I informed my supervisory ministry. Immediately, we informed the national health crisis committee, which convened an emergency meeting. A mixte investigative mission composed of menbers of the World Health Organization (WHO) and of the Ministry of Health was sent to the field on February 14, 2014. This mission carried out the first investigations on February 18. Its members realized the seriousness of the situation, faced with many deaths in the targeted localities. Professor Lamine Koïvogui, who was the head of the hemorrhagic fever laboratory within the team, called me to tell me that he suspected a viral hemorrhagic disease. He suggested not to wait for the end of this investigation, two weeks later, and to do everything possible so that we could send samples abroad to find out the exact origin, since he suspected hemorrhagic fever, probably Ebola. We were very concerned about this news.

The Doctors without Borders (MSF) office in Guinea mobilized all the means in its possession to help us send the samples on February 18 to France, precisely to Lyon, where Professor Celvin Benz's team was able to demonstrate the exact origin of this disease, which was indeed the Ebola virus, as early as February 21, 2014. This was very sad news for the country because it was the first time that the presence of this virus was mentioned in Guinea. Everyone thought it was a Central African disease.

We did not know how this disease could have migrated to Guinea. Nevertheless, since it was a case of a fatal disease, the WHO, according to the rules of surveillance, recalled that a statement had to be made, not only to the national community, but also to the international community. The first epidemic declaration was done by our Minister of Health, Colonel Remy Lamah, on March 23, 2014, to the people of Guinea and the international community.

Following this declaration, we reactivated the national health crisis committee. A first response plan was developed and submitted to the different partners. At that time, as the disease was concentrated in Guéckédou and Macenta, we really thought that we could control it within three to six months.

We benefited from training and information meetings in Ghana where the WHO gave us the broad lines to undertake the response to such an epidemic, based on basic strategies which consisted in organizing the surveillance of cases, not only to identify them, but also to follow up on contacts and samples, to transmit them to the laboratory to identify their cause to confirm or deny the initial diagnosis.

It was now necessary to organize the management of the cases. We couldn't admit them to the hospital, we had to build isolation centers specifically for them. This is how the concept of an Ebola treatment center was born and received all of the first cases, thanks to the support of Doctors without Borders, an NGO specialized in such treatment. Afterwards, we organized social mobilization and communication to inform the population, through our messages on prevention measures and knowledge of the disease itself, and organized logistics to enable our teams to transport not only the inputs needed for management, but also to carry out supervision missions and epidemiological investigations. We have also set up a "finance" committee in charge of mobilizing financial resources and managing them. There was also a coordination meeting set up at the national and decentralized levels. It was this meeting that established the foundations of the response.

Alas, despite these significant efforts, by the end of 2014, the number of cases was only increasing. We set up a coordination cell, endorsed by the government on September 5, 2014. I was appointed by the President of the Republic, coordinator of the response.

Afterwards, an inter-ministerial crisis management committee, was set up under the leadership of the Head of State, who was the first commander-in-chief of the response. The national health crisis committee had a somewhat marginal work, since the response was very specific instead of being transversal to all epidemics and disasters, and even environmental crises. The established cell dealt only with the Ebola epidemic.

Since I was the head of the surveillance commission, I was promoted to this position because at the beginning, we had set up commissions according to the strategies. There were four main commissions: treatment, logistics, surveillance, and a social mobilization.

The surveillance commission was responsible for collecting data in the field, establishing the evolutionary trends and the actual spread of the disease according to localities. The care commission was in charge of the isolation of living cases. As for the deceased, their dignified and secure burial was ensured by the Red Cross. We managed in this way until the coordination cell was born on June 5, 2014. Within it, were several units: logistics, communication, treatment, dignified and secure burials and security, following security problems for our intervention teams on the ground. The Pita building in the Chemin-de-Fer City was chosen as the coordination cell headquarters. We occupied the whole right wing. The fight was organized, and we lost health care workers to the disease in the affected prefectures. There was a prefectural coordination in Guéckédou and another in Kissidougou, with which we organized teleconferences every morning to know the situation and to take operational decisions. We remained in this mode until the end of 2014, only to find that our efforts were not up to our expectations, as the number of cases continued to increase. At first, only two prefectures were affected, but then five. In Guéckédou, those who attended the funeral of the director of the hospital in Macenta, who died of the disease, began to develop the same symptoms two weeks later. Unfortunately, a patient traveled and introduced the disease in the prefecture of Dabola, where some of our health workers lost their lives.

The five affected districts were Conakry, Nzérékoré, Dabola, and the two districts initially impacted.

With the plan that we had drafted, we had mobilized resources, but only theoretically since they could not be rapidly made available. When I say resources, I am referring to financial resources, material resources, and consumables needed for the fight. Three months passed between the announcement of financing and the availability of the funds, which curtailed the impact of our efforts in the field.

Besides, there was a delay in WHO's analysis, that did not immediately declare the disease to be a health emergency of international concern. There were fluctuations when the number of cases began to rise to the point of affecting Liberia and Sierra Leone. It was because of this escalation in the number of cases that the WHO eventually declared a health emergency of international concern. This resulted in WHO visits, and many personalities came to Guinea expressing their solidarity with our people.

What was very embarrassing was that Guinea had been subject to border closures. Only Mali did not close its borders with the Republic of Guinea. Many airlines suspended their flights to Guinea, except Air France and Air Maroc, which continued to fly to our country, so much so that our Head of State, Pr. Alpha Condé, said in one of his speeches: "Let's isolate the disease, but let's not isolate Guinea", thus calling for international solidarity.

It was in the months of November-December 2014 that we experienced the peak of the disease, more than 500 confirmed cases in a single month when until then we averaged 50. Our health centers became saturated. It is the lack of knowledge of the disease that caused this increase.

At the time, we did not know much about Ebola in Guinea. Its mode of transmission was not understood. Our customs and practices also contributed to the spread of the disease in Guinea, starting with the way people handle the body of people who died from Ebola. People washed the clothes of the deceased and came to greet other family members by shaking their hands. It was during these funerals that many people caught the disease and then served as a spreading vector to other communities. Warning messages were taken too lightly. People did not wash their hands with soap after outings. Standard preventive measures were not followed by some of our citizens. Messages were misinterpreted by many. Some were in denial, saying that it was imported by white people to Guinea. For some believers, it was a curse from God. These different interpretations led people to behave inappropriately, thus promoting the spread of the disease. To this day, some people still do not believe this disease exist, despite all the damage caused and the many deaths. These factors delayed our results on the ground. Furthermore, the available means of control were not really effective in cutting the chain of transmission.

In January 2015, inspired by our mistakes, we took new initiatives to control the disease. We designed a strategy based on awareness considering all the rumors and different interpretations. We orchestrated a community offensive coupling the active search for cases with an awareness campaign. We went door-to-door in the families and affected localities. We raised awareness, not only with posters and flyers, but also by asking inhabitants if there knew anyone who met the case definition. This new approach allowed us to detect new cases, and quickly isolate them for treatment. Some families, fearing that their relatives would be quarantined, hid them outside the village. This is how certain cases present in families escaped investigation. Nevertheless, this strategy allowed us to isolate nuemrous cases and reduce the burden on the country.

Prejudices led families to hide their sick loved ones outside the village. Fetishists and marabouts claimed to be able to cure this disease. We, who were able to really treat them were seen as spreading the virus! These prejudices caused some patients to flee from us and to undergo other treatments that wer not appropriate. After analyses, we were able to draw from our experiences the real reasons for the reluctance of the population to act and change their behavior. Some localities forbade access to our teams, which experienced violence and even deaths. This was the case in Womey, in the forest region.

The tragedy that occurred there was relayed by the media and other communication channels. Faced with interpret-tations that contradicted our interventions, we organized two successive meetings called "sacred union". The union concerned the entire population, civil society, political parties, religious leaders, and partners, who met so that we could stand together against Ebola rather than weaken ourselves in our fight against the disease. Fortunately, they all responded favorably. This was a turning point in the fight against Ebola in Guinea. Then, we put in place a new strategy called "Zero Ebola in 60 days.

With this strategy, we used returned nationals to lead community mobilization. We took the example of certain communities, notably Télémilé, Siguiri, Koyamah, on the Macenta side, who contributed to the control of the disease in their respective localities by sending nationals who helped in the sensitization, by bringing food aid to the villagers and by preventing other people coming from the affected localities from returning, to respect the isolation period of 21 days. Some even said: "No condolence addresses until the end of the containment period. We can call each other on the phone but no physical visits". Based on this, we described the "Zero Ebola in 60 days" strategy. Most of the localities were able to control the disease in less than 45 days instead of 60 days. This strategy allowed us to reduce the number of reluctant localities from 27 sub-districts to 4.

But, despite the effectiveness of this strategy, new cases continued to be reported in some districts.

In February 2015, the WHO proposed a vaccine called Merck that the government of Guinea welcomed. It was the first time that this vaccine was tested on a large number of people. After mechanisms were in place, on March 7, we started administering the vaccine.

I agreed to receive the vaccine so that my commitment to the fight would be a sincere commitment. It was a way to set an example for the people of Guinea. This vaccination was covered by the national and international press. I explained that I was motivated to receive this vaccine to silence doubts and as a mean to silence doubts and eradicate the disease in my country. This courage has been the subject of much discussion because a new product can have the opposite effect and even lead to death. As this was a trial, I had to sign a consent form in case something bad happened, that I would not be able to sue anyone, and that I would assume the consequences myself. I signed it. Some were for it and some against. When my family heard of it, my poor mother cried. She said that I had sacrificed myself for the country without her consent. It was the same with my wife. At that time, I had a very difficult time with my family. I was not in the same frame of mind as they were. My wife never shared my decision. I saw the mission I had been given as a duty. I was driven by faith and a sense of optimism. I knew that this product could serve me well. I got through that period of uncertainty, despite my diabetes, which was out of control. I had a bit of a fever, but after a few days, I regained my balance. Finally, this vaccine introduced our strategy, called "ring strategy".

At the same time, Liberia had succeeded in controlling the disease through strict containment of certain localities. The same strategy was proposed to Guinea. We went to visit Sierra Leone. It consisted in putting ropes around the concessions, delimiting the zone outside of which the inhabitants could not leave. This strategy was not applicable in Guinea, given the characteristics of our population. In addition, 2015 was a somewhat turbulent year, as it was an election year. We had to find an acceptable approach for the population. This is how this approach was born, which, instead of strict containment, favored a ring approach, which is a shared and accepted isolation. We therefore began by talking with the people to get their impressions. We sent a commission to the localities to speak with the inhabitants so that they would agree not to travel outside the circle of their village except in case of special exemption. They also had to agree to be visited in the morning and evening for temperature monitoring. Before agreeing to this, the villagers made a number of requests: to let their children go to school, to let them work their fields, and to give them food. Blocking them from going about their daily lives, we have to provide food. They also asked that we cover their health needs. During the

21 days of isolation, if someone got sick, he or she had to be treated for free. In exchange for this contract, the communities agreed to isolate themselves in return. At the same time, vaccination for all began. This is how Ebola was controlled in Guinea.

I will now start another chapter regarding the social perception and interpretation of the Ebola epidemic in Guinea. The way the people conceived of this disease and the way we conducted the fight were different. There was no symbiosis between us. We recognize that we were very normative at the beginning. Guided by the WHO guidelines, we followed an approach that showed its limits. We could not ignore the habits and customs and the perception of the communities. This explains to some extent the difficulty to control the disease at the beginning. There was no marriage between the health care team and the community, which was reluctant, which made interpretations, based on rumors, which led to fear and unnecessary deaths. I'll tell you a couple of anecdotes.

A Guinean man got into a cab but could not afford to pay the fare. When he got off, he said he felt like vomiting, that he was from Guéckédou and that he had Ebola. The driver saw the guy vomiting. Immediately, driver and passengers ran away. The guy quietly got out of the car and continued on his way without anyone daring to claim the fare.

Another man came to the BICIGUI to withdraw money. Faced with a long line, he asked: "Do you know where the toilets are? I come from Gueckedou; I need to go." People immediately fled, and he went to the counter to calmly take his money.

The third story happened here at our office at the National Health Security Agency. One of our health agents had died of Ebola and whose family had completed the 21 days of isolation. The State, with the support of the World Bank, had decided to give ten thousand dollars to the families of health workers who had died from the disease. The widow came to the agency. She was pregnant and our elevator was broken. When she got to the top of the stairs, she threw up, and people screamed. The citizens and even some experts said that Ebola was inside the Ebola coordination. That day, the "fighters" all fled. When my treatment expert told me this, I said, "If you doubt her, send her to the hospital, we'll examine her. She has completed the 21 days without symptoms, so if she is vomiting, it might just be because she is pregnant." The test was negative. To make fun of the run-aways, I wrote on social networks that pregnant women should no longer vomit in the public places at the risk of being taken for Ebola suspects, because experts fled from a pregnant woman who had vomited at the coordination. All this shows you a little bit the emotions created by Ebola.

More serious rumors circulated as well, including one that accused the "commander in chief" of sending the disease into the country with the help of accomplices. All of these rumors slowed our momentum in the fight against Ebola. The psychological state, the perception and the commitment of the population are very important in the fight against an epidemic. How can a population imagine that its president imported a disease into the country he leads? This is absurd! In my opinion, this is due to the fact that in African countries, people are too superstitious and sometimes skeptical. For example, in the villages, many of our grandfathers and grandmothers were accused of witchcraft, which naturally was not true. As soon as a child has a malaria attack, has convulsions, people automatically think that the child is being harassed by an old woman. It is a problem of mentality and false beliefs. I was once asked the same question and I answered: "How can you import a virus in a container from one country to another? ».

To this day, we still do not know where the first case came from and how the disease appeared, nor why in Guinea. No investigation has been able to pinpoint the origin of the virus. Rumors fed by people of bad faith wanted to tarnish the image of the head of state; 2015 was an election year. All these fallacious arguments were to disturb the national opinion about this situation. Nevertheless, after the two "sacred union" meetings, tension decreased.

The Wame massacre was caused by rumors. The Words can become weapons and cause much damage. How can one attack people who were simply there to raise awareness? The N'zérékoré governor with a health delegation, a security service, and members of the press had gone to sensitize the inhabitants of Wamé to the preventive measures that had been enacted to prevent the disease. The city of Nzérékoré itself was affected by the epidemic. Unfortunately, the inhabitants, under the influence of a rumor that these people had come to contaminate their locality, set up a lookout in front of the delegation. They blocked the road and came to attack them during one of their sensitization meeting. The first to suspect that the attackers were coming managed to flee in time with their reactive drivers. Unfortunately, during this attack, eight people died, eight people who were cut up and buried in a mass grave, due to the weight of rumors and prejudices about the disease. The authorities conducted investigations, the perpetrators were prosecuted, some were arrested and juged. But since we are in Guinea, the village elders came to convey their compassion to the government, and there was finally reconciliation with the sub-district of Wamé, which promised never to repeat such a tragedy. This is how this affair happened. This is the price paid for rumors. Personally, as a coordinator of the struggle, this act affected me a lot. Among the victims were close friends. The Prefectural Director of Health was a classmate and Deputy Director General of the hospital. I felt a lot of remorse following this despicable act. I could not understand that trying to save lives, they could cause the population to kill and cut human beings into small pieces. Unimaginable horror. In my heart, I keep this sad memory from the fight against Ebola in the Republic of Guinea.

Before Guinea, Ebola existed in rural areas in Congo-Kinshasa, but migrating to large cities was a first. The Head of State called upon a Congolese doctor, Dr. Jean Vivier Momboli, who came to advise the coordinator that I was. Through this man we benefited from the Congolese experience in managing Ebola in Congo. But he was quickly overwhelmed because in their country, Ebola occurred in small hamlets in rural areas. It was easier to control the situation in rural zones than in densely populated cities like Conakry or Guéckédou. Dr. Momboli learned many things in Guinea, because no two epidemics were ever the same.

A lot of measures had been taken, but the whole population and even the health workers and decision makers were overwhelmed by emotion. Everyone was in a state of emotion. We wanted to take drastic measures that were not applicable. For example, we wanted to isolate the first districts, Guéckédou and Macenta, and by extension the whole of Guinea-Forestière, but we realized that this type of isolation would be costly and perhaps ineffective. We therefore reviewed our strategies with measures that are acceptable to all and affordable. The coordination itself was very difficult to manage; setting up an interministerial committee, coordinating the information interpreted here and there, and having a single contact person were difficult. One of the negative effects of Ebola was the cancellation of Muslim and Christian pilgrimage, something that outraged Guineans. There was a lot of negotiation about this decision. This is one of the serious consequences of this disease. I will elaborate on the lessons learned in later chapters.

I have just evoked the emotional aspects of the struggle. Even health workers were afraid of the disease. Two hundred-fifteen doctors were infected, 115 died. There was fear everywhere, and stigma as a result. Some people who were declared healed were rejected by the population. Some agents were evicted from their homes by their landlords because of the disease.

People with Ebola often thought they were going to the hospital to be killed. The treatment failures have greatly affected our image in the fight. In Guéckédou, for example, where over 80% of patients died, people began to show their distrust. It is human. Imagine, someone sends a patient to the hospital and discover the body a short time later. That is a bit suspicious, isn't it? If it was one or two deaths, you could understand, but so many could lead to interpretation. False accusations circulated about our agents. People said that Doctors without Borders came to finish off the sick. This type of interpretation was very counterproductive in the fight against Ebola. Very often, people would threaten our treatment team. This was very difficult for me to understand, but people panicked because of the high mortality rate before we mastered treatment techniques, that is, to ensure that people are detected early. This is what the population interpreted to our disadvantage before coming back with better feelings later.

Here is a scenario that happened in 2016 during the resurgence in Koropara, a sub-district 80 kilometers from Nzérékoré. When we arrived in Koropara, many people went in hiding. We tried to find out why and discovered that the population thought we were coming to take their blood and organs to sell them in Europe. We invited the local elected officials and I told them how we had arrived by helicopter. I told the people that to come to Koropara, we were all weighed this morning. I told them we had three Europeans on the team. Among the Guineans who were in the helicopter, I was the one who weighed the most with 80 kilos. The European weighed 110 kilos and his Franco-American compatriot, Professor Pierre Rolin of CDC, weighed 120 kilos. I told the priest and the imam that if the Europeans had to look for the blood of Africans, it was better to use the blood of healthy people, especially those who weighed more than 100 kilos, to be able to draw blood from them without having any problems. They were the most suitable to have more vitamins than the rest of us who do not have access to the food they eat. That myself, I weigh more than all the villagers and you who are a chief who do not reach 60 kilos, so why would they need your blood and leave those? This made people laugh and that's how I was able to break the mistrust that was between us and the communities. Each of us spoke to explain the purpose of our mission and ask for their acceptance of our interventions. They opened their doors, and we were able to count the contacts, isolate them and even vaccinate them. Even the mayor, the officials, the governor, and the Prefect were vaccinated in front of them to show them that it was a good medicine that could help them. This acceptance allowed us to control the disease, whereas the first three days, they refused to accept us, even to the point of chasing away the first delegation.

Prejudices were such that there was a massive rejection of our team. During several interventions, I told the people of Guinea that I had not studied medicine to decimate them, and that I was a human being. I had a family, children, and under any circumstances could I play this terrible game. I told them that I was a believer and that after a pilgrimage to Mecca, I could never kill a person for any reason. I asked the detractors to beware of divulging bad information, because everyone will be accountable for what they say. Throughout the struggle, I tried to do enough communication to reduce the weight of prejudice. We even created mobile community radios and distributed solar radios to people so they could understand our actions. This allowed us to get people on our side to defeat this disease.

When an Ebola patient died, one of our teams took care of the body preparation, then put the body in a transparent plastic bag and during the burial, and the relatives could attend the burial by keeping a distance of 10 meters. As soon as we modified some of our measures and took into account the customs, they respected the measures and we ended up having their trust. At the beginning, by being too professional, we hurt the sensitivity of people. But we put things into perspective as we progressed in the fight.

Ebola is a disease that is clinically invisible to the naked eye but manifests itself primarily as fever and muscle pain. In the late stage, there may be vomiting and bloody diarrhea. But what was killing people was the bleeding. Ebola is a haemorrhagic disease where up to 30% of the subjects had internal bleeding and when the bleeding was intense, blood could come out of the mouth and nose. It is a disease with a very high mortality rate. In Guinea, Ebola killed 6 out of 10 people, whereas COVID-19 does not even kill 1% of sick people. In terms of mortality, Ebola is much more serious than COVID-19.

After Ebola, in early 2019, a case of Lassa Fever broke out in Kissidougou. We then had cases of yellow fever, a disease that killed many in Guinea. Apart from Cholera, these are the three diseases that have caused the most victims in our country. But if we take the number of victims in absolute terms, malaria is at the top of the list in terms of deaths in our country. Other diseases come and go, and their case-fatality rate is much higher than that of malaria, but they are not continuously present like malaria. For every 100 malaria cases, there are only one or two deaths, whereas for every 100 Ebola cases, 60 die. With Lassa fever, the mortality rate is around 20 out of 100 people.

I was asked if Ebola will ever come back. To say that Ebola will not return to Guinea is being overly optimistic. Ebola has its own cycle in different countries. When we look at the Democratic Republic of Congo (DRC), we see that the disease is still there, whereas before it could go five years without coming back. Let us pray to God that Ebola does not return to Guinea but as it came back to DRC numerous times, it is possible that it will be back here. In medicine, it is unwise to believe that a disease that has been fought once will not come back again. We have to be ready for the next occurrence and not be surprised by it. What remains clear is that if Ebola does return, it will not cause as much damage as it did the first time because we are now stronger and better prepared. We have learned. We have a vaccine, laboratories to diagnose Ebola, treatment and isolation centers, and trained agents to stop the disease. It will not be able to kill as many people in our country. When Ebola first came, we did not have a laboratory to diagnose it, so we had to send the first case (sample) to France to identify the disease. Today, we have 7 to 10 laboratories that can detect it in Conakry, in Nzérékoré, in Boké, in Kankan, in Guéckédou, etc. These techniques of prevention against Ebola are not taught in the universities of our country. In medicine, they teach classical medicine based on infectiology and general epidemiology. We have professors who pass on this knowledge, but they are didactic courses. It is with master's degree in public health that we get into the operational details. I have candidates in training who have participated in some of our investigations. They visited our museum. Only those who complet a master's have this possibility because it is a specialty for them. They are generalists. When you have to specialize, you have to know this most common diseases.

To get back to the history of Ebola, I think I've covered it all. There remains another aspect that I now want to address: the problematic of the management of human and material resources in the fight against Ebola.

The problematic of human resources management

During Ebola, there was a period of fear of the disease. We felt isolated in terms of support and human resources, to such an extent that, when the disease occurred in Guekedou, some partners went there, but the situation was considered very critical.

When I talk about partners, I mean NGOs and UN agencies. However, no agent from the central level of the Ministry of Health came to support the decentralized level of the Prefectural Health Directorate (DPS). The prefectural director of Guéckédou, who had never managed such an epidemic before, was herself very afraid of the disease. She notified me and asked for support from the central level. So, we organized a meeting at the Ministry of Health, looking for volunteers to go to Guéckédou. The choice was difficult with the echoes from Guéckédou perceived as a huge morgue.

I want to pay tribute to Dr. Pépé Bilivogui, who, unlike others whose names I prefer not to mention, spontaneously agreed to go. I told the Minister of Health that if no one wanted to go there as the primary surveillance officer, I would volunteer to go. He said, "If you go, who will stay in Conakry? I told him, "Wait, I will continue the consultation". Dr. Pépé Bilivogui who considers me like his brother said: "Wherever you send me, I will go. Because I know that you can't send me to a place where I can't serve.

So, he went to Guéckédou where he spent three months. He rendered honorable services to the Republic of Guinea and to the coordination. At the same time, of the partners who came to Guinea, 90% stayed in Conakry for the management of the crisis. We organized meetings. There were 200 or so of us and when meetings ended, they went to bed in hotels.

I would like to take this opportunity to pay a well-deserved tribute to the President of the Republic. When he realized that these experts were not in the field, he called for international solidarity for Guekedou, asking them to go and fight on the front line rather than rest in the hotels of Conakry. Several agencies responded to this call and the front lines began to have many human resources.

But coordination between the NGOs and the field agents was very problematic. Each organization wanted to work vertically with their flag, which sometimes led to differences of opinion and conflicts between partners.

At one point, there was over 104 vehicles in Forécariah. And in Koropara, when our teams arrived, the sub-prefecture that had never seen such an influx of vehicles, more than 40 vehicles in a sub-prefecture. Coordinating agencies and NGOs working in the same area of response was a real challenge. I want to underline how much effort we had to put in. Everyone wanted to work under the banner of the institution to which they belonged. We had to divide the country into zones because it was not easy to put certain partners together.

As for materials, it is true that we had a lot of support, but often the materials sent did not correspond to the real needs of the field. Some were never used. The situation was worse in terms of financial resources. And to this day, even I, as the person most responsible for the fight against Ebola, still do not know the exact cost of the response to Ebola. Some partners were not transparent. There have been pledges on which use we did not have visibility. There was opacity around financial management. All of these are problems constitute a problematic to improve on in the future. For example, some of the purchases made were "image boxes", but we had not taken into account the habits of the country. The paper culture did not exist, so we did not achieve the expected effects and wasted resources unnecessarily.

In terms of human resource management, we used a lot of people who did not do us any favors. The technical support we received was often for short stays of about two weeks. How to act in two weeks? How to benefit from their experiences in two weeks? Some also sent people who did not have enough knowledge to deal with the problems we were facing. Others came more to learn from us than to help us in the struggle.

On the Guinean side, there was not much enthusiasm at the beginning. Nevertheless, I would like to thank some young people, among the first hundred, whose help was invaluable. They were young volunteers who answered the call of the Head of State who also called on all retired health workers to mobilize for the fight against Ebola. Some of them, such as Dr. Facinet Yattara, volunteered to support us in the fight against Ebola. These were difficult times when we had no resources, not even the cost of transportation for these young people who came forward.

The second phase started with the arrival of funds, which made it possible to increase staff. In total, the technical staff involved in the fight reached 22,000 people. The Red Cross mobilized more than 8000 young people involved in all localities for the Ebola response. However, it is difficult to say exactly how many people were mobilized in this struggle. At one point, several returned nationals, all the ministers and even political leaders were mobilized. Returning nationals from villages were anonymous heroes throughout this struggle.

After the initial financial difficulties, Guinea was able to mobilize many resources. After Ebola, we were even able to save funds that allowed us to strengthen our health system. More than 36 Ebola treatment centers were built; health centers were upgraded with modern equipment. Boreholes were drilled not only for villages with Ebola patients but also for hospitals. Practically every hospital in the country had a borehole drilled with these funds. There was a lot of human resource trainings. Laboratories were put in place. We acquired invaluable resources through the rigorous management of Ebola funds. These same leftover Ebola funds allowed us to start the fight against COVID-19, which began in December 2019.

In summary, this is what I wanted to communicate about this topic.

Isolation and solidarity, a problematic equation ?

In this chapter, I will discuss the problem of epidemics and the fear it generates, and the reflex of affected and unaffected countries.

Guinea has been a victim of a rejection reflex. A Guinean student went to Senegal, after having been at this mother's side who some time later died of Ebola. Upon arrival in Senegal, his mother died of Ebola. Investigations around the case were able to identify among the contacts her son who had left for Senegal for his vacations from school. that the child had been with her for the last 15 days. Through the WHO, the Senegalese authorities were informed. The authorities found the student in treatment for malaria in a health center. Later, biological exams revealed the presence of Ebola. This news triggered a strong reaction from the Senegalese authorities who decided to go as far as closing the border with Guinea. Many returning Guinean were also victim of rejection because of suspicion.

In another case, a Guinean went to Mali following a mixed marriage between a Guinean and a Malian woman. When the Guinean man died of Ebola along with other family members, his wife was isolated and rejected. When she came to Nzérékoré, she was isolated in Beyla. It was afterwards that she called on me to provide food support. I contacted an NGO in the area to support her. But her mother, having heard the death of her husband and several members of her family, came to get her daughter's child. The child crossed our border in a vehicle. A week after his arrival, he developed symptoms of Ebola. This also caused a lot of interpretations. There was even a cross-border meeting between Guinean and Malian authorities who thought that there had been a relaxation of health control requirements on the Guinean side and that this was the cause of the entry of Ebola in Mali. I, myself, told the story and asked who was to blame. The vehicle that was transporting them was controlled by both the Guinean and the Malian border agents. The child was in the middle of his incubation period, so it was not possible to detect the disease. So, whose fault was it? The marriage between the two? Was love that origin of this? I told them that instead of blaming each other, it would be best to join hands to put out the fire. Finally, fraternity and solidarity prevailed on the emotion of rejection. I collaborated with Professor Samba Ousmane Sow who was the coordinator for Mali. He even later became minister. We knew each other well before. We knew each other from the leprosy days. I later collaborated with many WHO Malian executives with whom I had attended many training workshops.

Finally, solidarity prevailed. Mali and Guinea are like two lungs in one body. I will end this chapter by saying that in the face of a crisis, people must help each other, because today the danger may be in one country and tomorrow the same danger may reappear in another. Solidarity is what is needed between people. We must learn from history and humanize our activities. It is solidarity that must take precedence over rejection.

Management of the Ebola Epidemic

To address the subject of the management of this disease, I will divide it into 2 phases: first, the technical management that affects the epidemiological part and the second on the management of material, human and financial resources made available to us.

On the technical level, the first step was to reactivate a certain number of mechanisms. As soon as the epidemic declaration was made on February 23, 2014, the national committee of health crises activated the various commissions, namely: the surveillance commission, the treatment commission, the social mobilization commission, the logistics commission, and the coordination commission. The treatment commission included a sub-commission for dignified and safe burial that dealt with deaths. The surveillance commission also had a sub-commission, laboratory. Without a laboratory, the surveillance is blind!

At the beginning of the response, Guinea did not have a laboratory that could test for Ebola virus disease or a quarantine area to isolate such a disease. This delayed the implementation of some aspects of our technical guidelines. The laboratory problem was solved with the support of the World Health Organization (WHO), which sent a team from the Pasteur Institute in Dakar to validate and control the quality of the tests that were done in Guinea in the context of the epidemic. This team, mobilized by WHO, trained Guineans to enable them to identify the virus. Then, within the same framework of the laboratory, we benefited from the support of the French cooperation. Following a rise in cases, we received three Kaplan laboratories to support diagnostic efforts. We also benefited from a European laboratory based in Guéckédou that worked with Médecins sans Frontières to be able to follow up on the examination of hospitalized patients. The Russian Federation also participated in the diagnostic and management efforts in the Kindia prefecture. The United States also participated by donating a laboratory (DTRA).

Our first isolation center for patients was built in Guéckédou, the place where the disease was first detected, thanks to the support of French and Belgian Doctors Without Borders who combined their efforts to be able to make these centers available to us. A second center was built in Conakry and another in Macenta, to mention a few. Later, we also received the support of the United States Center for Disease Control and Prevention (CDC) which negotiated the establishment of the DTRA laboratory. CDC is an organization that covers not only the United States but also about sixty countries in the world with the Field Epidemiology Training Program (FETP). They came to Conakry from the very first hours to assist us with surveillance. They strengthened our laboratory capacity in Conakry. Multiple partners and countries provided assistance to Guinea in the areas of surveillance, contact tracing and social mobilization. In all, we counted 53 partners who contributed to the fight against the epidemic in the Republic of Guinea.

From March 2014 to December 2015, we set up the different commissions and teams. The national coordination for the Fight against Ebola that coordinated and directed the fight, and that organized a daily meeting in teleconference with the actors based in Guéckédou was created on the 5th of September 2014. We shared daily results, challenges and made decisions. Together, we sent joint teams to the localities and wrote a daily bulletin to analyze the trend of the disease. We were beginning to benefit from the use of new technologies in data management with DHIS2, which greatly helped us to monitor the epidemic. Cross-border meetings were organized by WHO and CDC between Guinea and its neighboring countries (Senegal, Mali, Liberia, and Sierra Leone), which allowed exchanges between the different teams and reinforced the spirit of sharing and solidarity.

During this phase, our main challenges were around resources because between the development of our first plan and the acquisition of resources, it took some time. The WHO also delayed declaring Ebola an international health emergency at the time, to the point that some people felt that people were not taking the magnitude of the disease into account based on what was actually happening on the ground. It is only after the declaration that the international community increased its visits to Guinea and affected countries. The declaration envigorated the fight against Ebola on the ground.

We developed budgets but some of the funds did not come until the end of the year. There was a huge delay, but I want to thank some of the partners who were there, WHO, UNICEF, Doctors Without Borders, and many others, who reprogrammed some of the funds they had in programs in Guinea, to redirect them to the fight against Ebola. That's what got us going in the beginning of this fight against the disease.

This was a initial handicap during the response. It is true that the government provided some initial funds to help, but not to the extent that was needed to fight the disease. We quickly realized that with these funds, we could only acquire the equipment that was in the country, but there was a need for many other materials that could only be purchased abroad: supplies, reagents and laboratory equipment, personal protective equipment, logistics, including even the means of travel between Conakry and Guéckédou by helicopter. It was necessary to be supported by external contributions. This is what was organized during the first period.

The other difficulty we had, we must admit, was that our established structures were not used to managing such an epidemic. Our meetings took too much time, sometimes 3 to 4 hours. We were late in making decisions and their implementation sometimes took more than a week, even though we were in an emergency situation. The availability of funds and equipment was delayed, which led us to think about solutions with the partners. Thus, a coordination was born on September 5, 2014, with the mandate to accelerate the provision of resources. I was appointed national coordinator.

Towards the end of the year, we noticed that there was much clumsiness in our messages. Some were even counterproductive, such as when we said we were facing a new disease with no known source and no effective medicine to fight it. This created panic among the population. When we communicated about preventive measures, including hand washing, and not touching bodies, it clashed with traditions. The way Guineans handle the dead, in the respect of customs and rites was forbidden, because it was a source of propagation of the disease. This caused conflict between our technical teams and the population, fed many rumors claiming even that the disease had been imported into Guinea with the complicity of certain authorities. In Africa, beliefs often carry a lot of weight. Some claimed that it was a divine punishment. Karamokos (diviners, marabouts) claimed that they could cure this disease. They even asked patients to refuse the treatments we offered!

This period was marked by many rumors and reluctance of the population to accept or accompany our interventions in the field. This resulted in an increase in the number of cases and the spread of the epidemic to other prefectures. By the end of the year, we found ourselves with more than twenty prefectures having reported cases of Ebola, including the capital, Conakry, where control was difficult.

The year 2015, brough the introduction of the Merck vaccine, in phase 3 of clinical trial, proposed by the World Health Organization (WHO) to Guinea. We studied the possibility of introducing it to interrupt the chain of transmission. Negotiations continued from January to February 2015, with the government authority having to make the political decision and the coordination having to, study the technical modalities for its implementation with the WHO. All inhabitants of the isolated locality were considered contacts and vaccinated. This ring vaccination strategy helped us to effectively control the disease in all identified households. Thus, we were able to declare the end of the epidemic in December 2015.

During this response many research studies were conducted, in particular: in the field of treatment with the use of Favipiravire, Interferon, Gelead, and plasma of the recovered, also in the field of vaccination with the Gamevac-combi of the Russian Federation, and the Merk vacccin (WHO). There were also studies on the serum of the entourage of the recovered, on the persistence of the virus in biological fluids including semen, and a vaccine trial (PREVAC) to study the combination of vaccines against Ebola, to determine the duration of immunity and their inocuity on children under 6 years of age by a consortium in Maféria.

After celebrating the end of the epidemic, we still had one area that had not been well controlled: the follow-up of Ebola survivors. Guinea counted a total of 1270 Ebola survivors, for which, with the level of knowledge at the time, was recommended 90 days of follow-up. We thought that after 90 days, it was impossible to transmit this disease and that the body would get rid of the Ebola virus. Many survivors were followed for those three months. At the same time, research was ongoing to see if the Ebola virus persisted in semen, as the Ebola virus is known to exist in fluids such as blood and vomit despite treatment. One study specifically mentioned the persistence of the virus in semen and showed fluctuations in this persistence. Some individuals who were completely negative, became slightly positive again after 2 to 3 months and then negative again and so on. Biologically, this showed us that the virus was hiding somewhere and that one day it could be the cause of a resurgence. According to the knowledge available at the time, the WHO considered that the risk of resurgence from cured subjects was practically infinitesimal, i.e. less than one case in a million survivors. In view of this, there was no follow-up program that exceeded three months. We continued to reinforce surveillance following the initial 42 days without any new cases.

In the first quarter of 2016, one of the Ebola recoveries, after 14 months, infected a contact in the prefecture of N'Zérékoré, specifically in the sub-prefecture of Koropara, which resulted in nearly eight deaths from Ebola. He did not show any clinical signs. Unfortunately, his wife died and other contacts caught the disease. This was a resurgence of the disease in a patient who became contagious again fourteen months after being declared healed. The hypothesis was now verified, the disease could reappear through one of these contacts.

The eight deceased were close relatives and those who participated in the washing of the bodies. It took a long time before the phenomenon was understood and detected, as, until then, it was considered very unlikely by the WHO. Our surveillance system was still working, but as Ebola was similar to malaria, when the first cases came to the health center, as we had declared the end of Ebola, the health worker did not suspect Ebola cases. It was when a cluster of deaths occurred that the prefecture became aware of the situation and began investigations. A sample sent to the laboratory confirmed the Ebola disease was back.

Unfortunately, a family member had traveled to Liberia, causing the disease to reappear there as well. He was identified and detected thanks to the good collaboration that exist between our two countries. This time, very quickly, the mechanisms to control the epidemic were put in place. Thanks to ring vaccination, in 45 days we were able to extinguish this new outbreak.

We have learned from this to strengthen our surveillance and diagnostic systems. I now want to share with you two anecdotes.

The first takes place in Koropara when the presence of Ebola was announced to the community. There was a lot of resistance against our intervention teams. Rumors are persistent. People were still afraid of Ebola, not only because of the high mortality rate, but also because of the residue of rumors that it was health workers who were spreading the virus. Many were opposed to our teams' intervention from the very first days. Fortunately, we quickly changed our communication strategy, which we had put in place around 2014. We quickly realized that we needed to integrate socio-anthropologists into the teams. Nevertheless, their approach required too much time. For example, when they gave us back the results of their surveys in Guéckédou, there were no more cases in the locality, and it was too late to apply their recommendations. I asked the socio-anthropologists to develop a different approach for emergency situations, based on the epidemiological difficulties identified and to work in collaboration with services in charge of surveillance and response to define their interventions. Until then, anthropologists chose their own themes of work. For example, they were looking for the impact of Ebola on female circumcision, whereas we were preoccupied with understanding the sociological bases that could explain the rejection of our interventions and rumors, and thus enable us to correct them.

Julienne Anoko, a Cameroonian socio-anthropologist who worked for UNICEF was the first to tackle the topic of resistance. One of her studies discussed why people were reluctant to put bodies in body bags. She looked for the socio-customary basis of this issue and this allowed us to understand the habits and customs and even to come to terms with the population, but also to change our strategy. From then on, we organized the body preparation and burial in the presence of family members, in order to silence the rumors that were circulating about the trafficking of organs taken from the deceased and sold in Europe. This is how the work of socio-antropologists has allowed us to get closer to the population.

The second case of this series of refusals and suspicion happened in Conakry. After this declaration of the end of Ebola, the response teams were reduced. When the disease occurred again, rumors spread, even among the authorities, that it was because we had reduced the response teams that the disease returned.

Faced with this exceptional situation, Pierre Rolin, who has followed more than 12 Ebola epidemics in Central Africa and throughout the world, immediately came from Atlanta (USA) to Guinea to investigate the reasons for such a phenomenon. The response team was quickly summoned to explain the real reasons for the resurgence of the disease, because it created a lot of emotion. As Pierre Rolin had a better grasp of the situation than any of us, he was our spokesperson before the Head of State who wanted to understand why Ebola had returned to the Koropara prefecture, in Nzérékoré. He certified that this was the first time Ebola had reappeared in a person who had been cured for fourteen months. Until then, assumptions suggested that it was no more than three months. He was there to figure out how this could have happened. Finally, he said that it had been possible through the semen, but the health authority had no information to suggest that it could persist in the semen of a survivor. Our health authorities did not have information that could have led us think that the disease could survive this long in the sperm and cause a resurgence. The scientific evidence won the heart of everyone and we were ordered to go to the site to do everything possible to ensure that this disease does not gain ground again from Koropara to other sub-prefectures. All means were put at our disposal.

The disease triggered a lot of emotions and interpretations. If the factual causes were not quickly elucidated by the technical teams, decisions made could interfere with our response momentum.

Other anecdotes involve patients who have recovered from Ebola. One family in Guinea was nearly decimated by Ebola with only three survivors out of nine infected people. I had to make a trip to Ghana with two of those survivors. We were invited by the Guinean ambassador to Ghana to a dinner. We were invited with the Minister of Health, Colonel Rémy Lama. When we were around the table, at dinner time, the ambassador asked that everyone introduce themselves, which was done. When I introduced the two people who were with me as Ebola survivors, I saw the ambassador's face change. He couldn't eat and told me he wanted to see me in private. He said to me: "Doctor, I invited you and the minister, why did you bring Ebola patients to my building? "I answered: "I myself traveled with these two people and we stayed together night and day. If there was a risk of being exposed, it would be us rather than you, who only receive them for a few minutes. They are completely healed. Even two months ago, they were tested and there is no longer any risk of them infecting anyone. He finally told me "Sakoba: you should have told me". And I told him that I was sorry and if we had to leave, I would go out with them because when your look changed, they were hurt in their souls. I'm sure after the meal they will notify me. I brought them to free them, to consider them also as human beings. They were told that they are healed so they can no longer contaminate others and are not a risk to our community. After this exchange, we continued to eat but his demeaner was a bit off. We also tried to cheer up the two survivors so we could continue the dinner. One of the two survivors was hired by Doctors Without Borders after being rejected from the treatment center where he worked. Doctors without Borders led the way in destigmatizing the disease. There was a lot of stigma attached to those who recovered from Ebola and the partners helped me afterwards to reconcile them with their communities.

Other rumor-driven events were reported in Faranah, where an MSF car was completely burned. Fortunately, there was only material damage and no loss of life.

Another incident occurred in Tanènè, in the Dubreka prefecture, where one of our contacts who had tested positive infected a family member. The ambulance had come to pick up the confirmed case to take him to an Ebola treatment center. This gentleman had prejudices against Ebola and thought that instead of treating people, we were killing them with injections. Because of the high lethality, people saw Ebola centers as places to die. This prejudice led this citizen to chase the ambulance to get his sister out of it and throw a bottle of gasoline inside to set it on fire. When the ambulance stopped, the driver and the nurse were beaten up. The nurse had to be hospitalized because of the violence he experienced. The sister of the attacker, whose care was interrupted, finally died. After this scene, the man was arrested but the rumors resulted in the lost of an ambulance, completely burned.

Finally, another situation took place in Yimbaya (Conakry) when we were attempting to set up an isolation center in each commune to reduce the distances to be covered when referring cases. The population of Yimbaya was reluctant. They saw the establishment of the center as a threat to their lives. For them, the center, instead of treating people, would contaminate their relatives. As the first person in charge of the coordination, I went there, supported by the French ambassador and other personalities, to convince the people of the need to set up a treatment center to facilitate the treatment of the sick in their commune. When we arrived, we very quickly noticed that the atmosphere was heating up between us and the young people, who were there to refuse the establishment of the treatment center. Personally, I tried to flee because a policeman had told me once that when the population is angry, you don't reason with them, you must leave the place until the tension subsides. So, remembering that, I tried to sneak away to avoid a bad ending. At the same time, the security services evacuated the French ambassador. We were all able to leave the place safely.

These scenes that occurred during the Ebola epidemic show us how emotions and rumors can cause danger within a community. It is now up to us to learn lessons to be able to manage these cases because these manifestations of refusal slow down our intervention on the ground. At times, this has led to much more violence than the epidemic itself, rumors killing more than the disease. Rumors are very dangerous viruses for the life of the community. It is time to find a solution to all these major epidemics, especially these new diseases, and to think about a strategy to combat the rumors that hinder interventions and cause deaths and destruction of public property.

In the management of Ebola, the difficulties are multifold. The first is the acceptance of technical guidelines by the actors and stakeholders. The first stakeholder for me is the community, no matter how good or strong our interventions are, if they are not accepted, we may not achieve the expected results. This is therefore countered by rumors and opinions. Therefore, we now advise conducting socio-anthropological studies and adapting interventions to the local context. In

Guinea, moreover, this mistake was made at the very beginning of the disease. We thought that the strategies that were recommended to us and that helped control the spread of the disease in Forest Guinea were applicable in Lower Guinea, some 600 kilometers away, even though the customs and habits are different. We even sent the entire team that controlled the disease to Guéckédou, to Forécariah, which had become the epicenter because the epidemic had migrated to the Lower Coast, in line with Kambiyah in Sierra Leone. These same teams encountered reluctance.

The second order was, at the level of the authorities at times, we had more than two million plans because every Guinean thought they had the best solution to control the disease. With these interpretations and perceptions, how do you get them to intervene in a much more rational and factual way? Most of the solutions we were offered were based on emotion and perception. It was not based on technical, factual aspects of problem solving. So, sometimes convincing certain authorities caused us problems and as they were the ones in charge of the sectors of health, agriculture, sometimes presidents of the committees of management of health crises in their localities, it was a challenge. Even at the governmental level, we had difficulties convincing them to adhere to our interventions which were based purely on technical considerations. Here again, management must reconcile the two, because one party must not feel excluded from the process. Everyone should know exactly what role to play to collaborate with the stakeholders. This was the second level of knowing how to manage all the actors.

With the technical actors, the biggest difficulty I had was how to get the technical actors to remove this image of each partner holding his flag and rather than working alone to work in synergy with others. In all, 53 partners were involved but 2/3 were technical partners in the field. We had difficulties in mapping the interventions and in professsionalizing them.

Surveillance was led by WHO and CDC because they are specialized in surveillance. MSF was the leader for the treatment of the disease because in our opinion, they were the most competent partner in this field. Social mobilization was led by UNICEF, to name a few. When the fight reached a certain level, many did not respect their field of intervention. They accumulated areas and funding, and programmed activities, creating interference between the partners to such an extent that UNMEER, which was in charge of the United Nations agencies, was forced to intervene within its own units. UNMEER was sent by the United Nations to Guinea, with a contingent of nearly 55 people to support the coordination of interventions. UNMEER was initially led by a man from Rwanda. Unfortunately, this man died in his hotel room at the Millennium in Guinea. To this day, the cause of his death is unknown. He was replaced by a Senegalese named Diop who led the rest of the epidemic until the end, with the occasional visits of David Navarro, who was appointed as the person in charge of the Ebola response to bring order. As he answered directly to the United Nations, he ensured the coordination of interventions and helped the local coordination to manage its interference. I personally spent a lot of time with other NGOs, of which there were many, to help manage the teams.

The other dark point of responses was a difficulty concerning the harmonization of the paiement of the recruited agents. Each partner had its own grid, the State also had its own grid, which created jealousy between the actors who played the same role but were not paid the same. The WHO used a grid with the highest pay, while those who were in care with Doctors without Borders had an average pay compared to the surveillance agents. Some of the young people knew this because their colleagues worked there.

They were the most exposed because they were working directly with the confirmed cases. They wanted to go on strike, and it took almost a month of negotiations before a solution was found, thanks to the World Bank, which agreed to provide additional funds for their salary to balance the salary problem.

The problem of managing partners in the different areas of intervention slowed down our response, not to mention that some of the experts present were not up to the task. At the beginning of the epidemic, there were more than 300 experts based in Conakry. At the time, the disease was in Guéckédou, and the Head of State made an announcement that he wanted the experts to go there. Only the agents of Doctors Without Borders and WHO were on the ground. After the announcement, each partner examined its situation and sent staff to Guekedou. This re-energized the response.

The last problem was financial management. We had taken considerable time to mobilize the necessary resources. We did not have an isolation center. The isolation centers that Doctors without Borders set up in Guéckédou and Conakry were quickly erected. It was hot inside, with patients vomiting. These were difficult conditions, and it was only later that we had more modern centers in Macenta and other localities, with air-conditioned rooms. Then, we were able to build centers dedicated to sick healthcare workers. We recorded 215 infected healthcare workers, 115 of whom died. Finally, thanks to the French Cooperation, we were able to build all of these centers that offered better conditions. Faced with the shortage of beds following the increase in the number of cases in Conakry, a new care center was also opened in Coyah with the support of a Cuban medical brigade. But all these constructions took time, imagine a disease declared in March, and many of these centers could not be finalized until late 2014 and some even in January 2015. This contributed to the delay in disease control and case management. These are lessons we need to learn, so that all can be in place before the occurrence of the next disease, which was actually the case when COVID-19 hit Guinea.

Two factors helped our teams to continue despite the challenges mentioned. The first factor is the team spirit that made it possible to maintain cohesion between us. The other factor is the trust of the Head of State, who took the lead of the response. My teams worked everyday to deserve his trust. Strengthen by his recognition, I felt very motivated and invested with a mission that led me to set an example by being the first to receive this vaccine on a trial basis. Despite the potential risks involved, I decided to be the first guinea pig. I could have had an anaphylactic reaction and even died, but I persisted. This motivation led me to set an example alined with my ideas. It was not obvious that the Guinean people would accept this vaccine at the time. The members of the coordination were divided; 50% were against it and the other 50% were for it. Among the partners, some were also against it. I'm not naming anyone here, but they were against the rollout of the vaccine. A Canadian vaccine was bought by the United States and made available to the WHO as a likely weapon to save humanity. This vaccine had not been tested on a large number of people in an epidemic situation. Guinea was the first country to test it. Although the first and second phases of the trial were fully completed, we contributed to the third phase. After us, DRC and Sierra Leone also used it. At the end of 2015 that there was a first publication in the *Lancet* journal indicating that this vaccine was safe and that it could be licensed. Now, things have evolved, the vaccine was approved by the American and European authorities in December 2019. It is indeed registered today as an effective weapon against Ebola.

The disease was moving progressively, from one locality to the other, but we managed to register some victories that motivated us in our fight. These small victories from prefecture to prefecture and from locality to locality were a very pleasant factor. Secondly, the team spirit was uplifting. I am very grateful to the contingent of young people who came to me following the call made by the Head of State, Professor Alpha Condé, inviting all health workers including retirees and those who are in office to mobilize to face this disease. When this first group arrived, we had no financial means of motivation, not even to feed these young people who had come to volunteer to save the country. This act was motivating because I felt that I was not alone in my commitment to saving lives in our communities. Many others came to the rescue of the nation. Of course, there were some elders, but the young people were the most numerous. They said to me: "Doctor, even if you are not here, we will be here to carry the torch". And these young people continued with me to lead the response against Ebola.

The other motivating factor was the support of the authorities in all our actions. Each time we had needs, the government tried to put means at our disposal and also to support us morally, so that we could continue the fight.

The fourth support that I really appreciated was that of my family because I had periods of discouragement in front of certain difficulties. My family, with my dear mother at the forefront, encouraged me from time to time to resist discouragement in order to deserve the confidence of the Head of State. I also had to hold press conferences where the people expressed their gratitude towards me.

The last factor is the satisfaction expressed not only by the partners but also by the components of my society in regard to the fight I was leading. This allowed me to resist the weight of fatigue and difficulties.

In this management, first, I would pay tribute to the victims among our collaborators who, while trying to save lives, lost theirs. We already talked about Womey and the 115 people who died in the fight, just like soldiers who died on the battlefield. I pay them a heartfelt tribute. I am grateful and pray to God that their souls rest in peace. Also, in general, I pay tribute to all the victims of Ebola because, in their loss we lost relatives and Guinean citizens who could contribute to the development of this country.

I pay tribute to the two international experts (Rwandan and Cuban) mobilized for the response who died in the Republic of Guinea, far from their families, from non-Ebola causes.

I pay tribute to my collaborators, whose list is far from exhaustive. Some of them have distinguished themselves and helped me in the coordination of this fight. From the beginning of the epidemic, the French cooperation sent several experts to support the coordination of the response. Among others, we can mention Professor René Migliani who stayed with me throughout the response and whose contributions were very significant for the control of this epidemic. He attended all our meetings with the Head of State to support the strategic and technical discussions. Through him, I thank all his compatriots.

Also, Dr. Roland Emmanuel Malano and Dr. Facinet Yattara came to me and said: "Doctor, I am coming to your aid to participate in the management of the response against this disease". Dr. Fatou Sakho, Dr. Moussa Konate, Dr. Moumie Barry and Dr. Momo Camara who, although he was secretary general at the Ministry of Health and retired, also said to me: "Doctor, send me wherever you want but I want to participate in this fight". The nomination of Dr. Sekou Conde to the position of deputy director of the National Cell for the Fight against Ebola was highly beneficial to the administrative and financial management of the response. He demonstrated competence and mastery of the procedures. Considering the urgency of our activities, an adaptation of these procedures was essential to reduce the delays in payment which negatively impacted the response at the beginning. The set up of accelerated procedures and considering the requirements of partners were not always easy.

The chief doctor of the coordination in Guéckédou who is very famous, Abdourahamane Batchily, led the victory in Forécariah. I must thank Dr. Pépé Bilivogui, whose story I have already told, for his courage because, at the time, it was not easy to find someone for this mission. The other person to thank and congratulate is the Minister of Health, Remy Lamah, who supported me and was ready to go to the front whenever the need arose, and the government authority was called upon. He provided this supervision and support. He is a military man by training and showed a sense of patriotism with the work with which was entrusted. Through him, I thank all the other Ministers, governers, prefets, sub-prefects, and members of the civil society, the national NGOs, the religious leaders, the associations of returning nationals, the journalists, the artists, the economic operators, and in particular the first lady of the country who invested herself in a very special way in this response.

I would also like to thank Mr. Baba Alimou Barry and Mr. Kassim Diare, both chief accountants, whose rigorous financial and material management largely contributed to the success of the response.

Some partners have distinguished themselves in this struggle. I am referring to the CDC experts, some of whom have distinguished themselves by the length of their stay and by their contribution, in particular Dr. Pierre Rollin, Dr. Benjamin Dahl, Dr. Michael Kinzer, and Dr. Lise Martel. From WHO, I am thinking of Professor Jean-Marie Dangou, Dr. Mohamed Belhocine, Dr. René Zitsameme Coddy, and Dr. Dyingarey. For Unicef: Dr. Mohamed Ayoya and Dr. Guy Wogo, without forgetting the numerous collaborators from MSF and the Red Cross, who conducted secure and dignified burials. In any case, as the first person in charge of the coordination for the fight against Ebola, I am grateful to them for a job well done. We were 52 people at the coordination. It is true that we could not all be decorated, but they all distinguished themselves. I am negotiating with the authority since 2015 so that all these people are officially decorated.

Ebola was the biggest battle of my life. I said in my speech at the end of the epidemic that despite my experience with more than 30 epidemics, mainly yellow fever and meningitis, I had never been confronted with so many emotions and difficulties. This epidemic caused as many deaths as other epidemics in Guinea, including cholera because the mortality rate of the latest did not exceed 5%. With Ebola, we reached 80%. The difference was monumental. Ebola created many problems, especially socio-economic ones, by paralyzing the health system. For example, once the crisis was over, Guinea had to deal with a major measles epidemic because children were no longer vaccined. Vaccination programs had been interrupted at the time of Ebola to limit the risk of transmission. Guinea paid the consequences of this drop in attendance at our facilities, some of which had been closed. This drop varied from 30% to 100% for some facilities. This is to tell you how difficult this period was.

Now, despite my experience having managed over 30 epidemics, and that I had often communicated in front of the press, it is Ebola that has brought me fame, nationally and internationally. I gave thanks to the President of the Republic who had confidence in me to put me at the head of this coordination and who allowed me to express a competence that I myself did not know I had. Like all men, it is often in certain situations that buried competences are revealed. I was very shy at school, and I remained so for a long time during my career, but today, thanks to this position of coordinator, I can express myself freely in front of an audience. I am often told that I communicate well, but I still need to listen to myself to be sure. I like to listen to great traditional speakers to improve myself. In particular, I listen to communcators, the imams and priests, to understand their rhythm and the way they convey their messages. Some Guinean and foreign politicians do not leave me indifferent either. I also learn through the internet how to conduct an effective communication. All this has allowed me to improve myself and to adapt my communication to the audience, in order to avoid being too technical when I address the population for example.

At times, during the Ebola epidemic, my communication sometimes caused some misunderstanding with authorities, who at times threatened to forbide me from communicating on sensitive subjects related to the problematic of managing epidemiological data, presented in weekly bulletins and press conferences.

I did not insist too much on the management of material resources, but I can say that much material resources were sent without a prior evaluation of needs, so that, after Ebola, we had a stock for which we had no use. We had laboratory equipment for which the reagents or tools are not accessible or are too expensive for the budget of the Ministry of Health. This provide lessons for the next epidemics, so that real needs are assessed to avoid buying items that cannot reinforce our health systems. In the future, we should take into account the opinion of technicians on the ground, avoid relying on partners or friends ordering according to their personal experience or what was used elsewhere, and take into account local expertise when ordering. I think it is being corrected with the COVID-19 epidemic. Having now the orders approved by the laboratory commission and other commissions reduces the waste of ressources.

Regarding finances, like I already said, to this day, I do not know the cost of the Ebola response. Certain partners managed funds but did not share their financial situation with us. The Ministry of Health put in place two principles: transparency and accountability. Many partners violated these principles even if we were not asking them to put their ressources under our control but simply informing us of the ressources that were given to Guinea. There were clashes. Nevertheless, on the positive side, with the efforts of the government and technicians, the epidemic did not last as long as anticipated, and some remaining funds could be used to not only reinforce the training of our health agents but also build some health infrastructure, mainly centers for the isolation of patients infected with an epidemic-prone disease. Thirty-eight certers were built and laboratories were equipped to provide local diagnostic confirmation. Some of the remaining funds were used to control measles between 2017 and 2019, and then to start the COVID-19 response.

This is how financial donations were used with the approval of our donating partners. I take this opportunity to invite all partners, from the beginning of an epidemic to respect the national directives of transparency and accountability. This positive consequence prepared Guinea for its fight against COVID-19.

Lessons to be learned

After any event, lessons are learned to prepare for future events. While Guinea was not the first country to be affected - several outbreaks were previously reported in the Democratic Republic of Congo, Congo-Brazzaville, and Uganda - this was the first time Ebola had occurred in the Republic of Guinea. It is also important to recognize that this was the first time Ebola became urban, attacking major cities like Conakry, Kindia, and Guéckédou. So, it was a new experience. An epidemic is never identical to another. We had to learn lessons so that from now on, we could correct the shortcomings that we had observed during the response.

In discussing the lessons to be learned, we will start with the technical aspects.

Technically, we quickly realized that we were not prepared for such an event that came as a surprise. We spent too much time highlighting the nature of the epidemic, which, according to subsequent investigations, started in Guinea around December 2013, but was only confirmed in March 2014. This lack of preparedness to diagnose the disease caused us a three-month delay when, in surveillance, any new event should be detected within 48 hours. Secondly, in terms of preparedness, the human resources did not have the competence to deal with such a disease. The Ministry of Health did not have the infrastructure to hospitalize all confirmed cases. Finally, financially, we did not have enough resources to manage such an event.

To return to the technical level, we had no laboratory capable to detect the disease, which meant that the first samples had to be sent to France. With this in mind, we initiated solutions to prepare Guinea for such an event in the future, which can occur at any time and in any country. At the beginning, we believed that Ebola was a disease of Central Africa and that it could not arrive in West Africa because no case had been recorded here in history, so that until now, people wonder how, from Central Africa, this disease could migrate to West Africa.

In terms of lessons learned, if the disease entered our country, it was due to a weakness in our health system. Even before the end of the epidemic, we identified these weaknesses and developed a capacity building program that we called "the resilience problem". Training was initiated for this purpose. Rapid response teams have also been set up. We have strengthened the capacity of our laboratories.

I think countries need to put special emphasis on health system preparedness and financing. We need to do more prevention than treatment in our health programs. Since emergencies are too frequent in our country, we must devote a significant part of the state budget to them so that we can reduce the negative effects on our health system by reversing the evolutionary trend of certain events that can surprise us and whose origins are very often unknown.

The Ministry of Health budget is below the requirements of the West African Health Organization (WAHO), which asked that 15% of our national budget be devoted to health. It must be recognized that Guinea has gone from about 2 to 3% to 8% in 2018. But we are still far from the figures hoped for or the quotas required by the OAS. It is therefore easy to understand why the health sector is underfunded.

Funding for emergency situations is also insufficient. ERARE teams emerged as a necessity. They were founded on the ashes of the prevention teams that existed in earlier periods and were responsible for surveillance and control of epidemics. But these teams were starved of resources. The vehicles and resources were no longer there. By the time Ebola came along, none of those teams in the interior of the country were functioning! I, myself, was the head of the mobile team in the Kankan region for about ten years. Since the 1990s, these teams were in place but dormant. The Ebola epidemic brought these teams back to life and they were renamed, with the assistance from the European Union and of Bioforce. Even the assignment of these teams was reviewed by the technical staff and the response specialists. We named them the regional alert and response teams (Acronym: ERARE in French), prepared for the treatment and detection of the disease in the prefectures under the respective regions. It was a good idea to strengthen these teams because they filled a gap in our response.

As for the conduct of the response, in general terms, here is what we can retain. With the advice of the United Nations services, notably WHO and UNICEF, as well as the CDC, we were quickly confronted with the problems of adaptation to our local realities. These major strategies, training and management, followed the WHO guidelines. But in public health, measures must always be adapted. We were obliged, in the face of various problems, to make this adaptation. Starting with coordination, the committee that was in place very quickly showed its limitations. We immediately set up a national coordination with a clear mandate. In short, we adapted our management structure as we went along, until we practically set up a parallel structure that depended directly on the coordination and had its representations at the level of the prefectures, which we called "prefectural response coordination".

This prefectural coordination managed the activities on site and the different prefects were the presidents of the monitoring and control body, which was the crisis committee at the prefectural level. This chain, which brought the intervention level closer to the strategic decision-making level, made it possible to carry out response activities in real time and to obtain results that we could share with various partners. In regards to the management of the response, we noted that we needed to strengthen the coordination aspects. The first challenge was to prepare the coordination and the strengthening of the teams in charge of managing epidemic emergencies. Since 2007, a decree had put in place these committees, but they were not functional at the time Ebola broke out. The biggest challenge was that in the interior of the country, there was no system to report to local authorities on the main health challenges that arose on a regular basis. It is essential that at the prefecture level, the authority, the prefect and his cabinet, be aware of the epidemiological situation in their prefecture without waiting for epidemics to occur. They must be provided with field data. However, this lack of collaboration exists in most of our prefectures where, often, those in charge are not aware of what is happening on the ground, in terms of health and epidemiology. In terms of infrastructure, they are involved in inaugurations and other events, but as for the evolution of diseases, they do not have an understanding. Concrete support from the health authorities is needed. At some point, at the prefecture level, there must be a kind of autonomy and visibility on the actions taken rather than just sending reports to the prefectural authority. The same goes for the national level. There should be a clear structure that provides information, through the Minister of Health, during inter-ministerial meetings, on the evolution of the situation at the national level and in relation to the epidemic.

I would like to salute the Head of State who followed the evolution of the Ebola epidemic on a daily basis. But this was not the case in the decentralized structures. This was a major challenge. The challenge in terms of preparedness is that the health infrastructure for these diseases with epidemic potential must be strengthened. The COVID-19 that we are experiencing now has very quickly shown our limits. But it is not just Guinea. Most countries were overwhelmed. I would like the country to have the capacity to rapidly deploy and erect alternative structures, such as tents, when needed.

There are educational challenges. There needs to be a system of continuing education to maximize the knowledge of medical staff. That is one of the things that needs to be improved. We also need to plan a program to strengthen our health system and address all the gaps that we saw during Ebola. We need to work with partners to take steps to strengthen our systems so that in the future we can prevent another Ebola-like event.

As far as areas for improvement are concerned, we can summarize this in a few words. First of all, in regard to continuing education, we need on-the-job trainings and academic degrees. In order to carry out certain analyses and forecasts and to develop plans, you need people of a certain level.

We also need to make improvements in laboratory equipment because we quickly realized that the equipment, we were using could not detect new viruses. Arrangements should be made to update our capacity to confirm the various diseases, and also to decentralize the diagnostic capacity. Only Conakry was able to conduct tests, which was very limiting for the other prefectures. We need to analyze the situation according to the road accessibility and decentralize the means of diagnosis by training the laboratory technicians accordingly, but not in one site only. The other challenge is equipment. Personal protective equipment for infection prevention and control was insufficient to meet the challenges. We need to minimize the exposure of our health workers to diseases. One of the points I will emphasize is social mobilization, taking into account the level of illiteracy in our country and the customs and traditions. It is always good, as part of the preparation, to involve the communities (with sensitization) to prepare themselves against epidemics, to teach people the different behaviors to follow and their role in the detection. This was not the case at the beginning of the response. It is only after a year that we were able to include community participation, give the community visibility and allow it to take the lead in our interventions. This is one of the points to improve. It is from this point on that socio-anthropologists were sent to the frontline to facilitate the relationship between the community and the intervention team.

At the preparedness level, a training module needs to be developed, such as "How do we help decision makers make good decisions?" We need policy makers to consult with technicians in making technical decisions about our prevention strategies. Decisions will need to be based on technical input from technicians, whether they are socio-anthropologists or epidemiologists. These decisions can be quickly implemented. Decisions that are not made on technical grounds often turn out to be unworkable. This is not good, especially in the management of epidemics.

After this epidemic, we developed a preparedness plan that we are currently implementing.

I mentioned the main points to be improved in terms of training, infrastructure, equipment, laboratory capacity building and also in terms of social mobilization and communication. A five-year plan is being implemented. There is a plan to strengthen the capacities of the national health security agency. It is in this plan that the Coordination of the Response against Ebola was dissolved. We decided to create in its place a permanent structure, which is now the National Health Security Agency (ANSS – French acronym), responsible for organizing data collection, surveillance, responses, and preparing the reinforcement of the country's capacity for health security. This plan is being implemented.

This Ebola outbreak has allowed us to learn a great deal about our environment from a socio-anthropological perspective. At first, while we used strategies guided by the

World Health Organization and the CDC, we then confronted local realities. What were the points of confrontation? The customs, and the treatment of our dead and their bodies. We had placed bodies in body bags that did not respect the social norms of our country. As a result, we observed much reluctance. The fact that we did not involve the socio-anthropologists led to rumors that we, instead of being people who helped them fight the disease, were criminals who spread it. Some of our partners were accused of being there to sell the organs of Ebola victims. Those were the rejection factors. The high mortality rate, which reached 80% at one point in the fight, created a crisis of confidence between the communities and us. Some sections of our society were using these problems to draw people to them. I am talking about traditional doctors and marabouts who said that modern medicine could not treat Ebola, but they could. So, people ended up thinking, well, since these doctors don't have a vaccine or medicine for Ebola, why would we go to the isolation centers? People's misinterpretation was a limiting factor. This delayed the management and evolution of the response because the communities did not buy into our control strategy at the time. This was a lesson and we realized that we needed to involve more socio-anthropologists to facilitate community understanding. We also realized that with any solution, it was necessary to involve opinion leaders, returning nationals, and influential men of the community to ensure their support of our solution or plan. Faced with these challenges, these are the solutions that we had to experiment with and that we will have to reinforce in the future, especially the involvement of leaders. Their involvement in the fight against Ebola has been very favorable for us because, as the Head of State said, the message is understood by the bearer of the message. The same message can be conveyed by several people, but if the bearer is not credible, the content of the message may be inadequate in its implementation. Therefore, we chose credible men, known in their environment, to involve them in the dissemination of the messages, in our interventions, which made that the places which were closed to us were opened as soon as we practiced this method. The prejudices that were circulating disappeared.

Other lessons include the need for traditional disease response strategies to take into account socio-anthropological factors to give us a better chance of producing good results. Guinea has paid a heavy price in terms of conflicts in our strategic interventions and social acceptance in the distribution of materials, up to and including the deaths of men during the Ebola epidemic. These are tragedies that we can avoid in the future, with better preparation, better community mobilization, and an effort in communication to resolve socio-cultural misunderstandings in the response and also to fight against rumors.

With regard to the future, Guinea has developed a communication plan that gives a decisive place to the intervention of socio-anthropologists and community leaders in our communication strategies. Training at this level has made it possible to integrate the community into the different levels of our intervention and to give them a role for a better understanding of our interventions by the communities. This has allowed us to approach the response during this new COVID-19 pandemic with ease.

From the point of view of collaboration, at the level of the partners, it was not always easy. One of the challenges was the divergence of views in the training and in the analysis of things. Each country has its own way of organizing responses to epidemics and has different structures. Each country approaches an epidemic differently. This technical misunderstanding was quickly expressed during our discussions and epidemiological meetings.

The second point is the mapping of interventions by area and location. Often, we had too many partners who have the same functions. It was very difficult to put together those who have complementary functions. This was a challenge when coordinating. It was not easy to put two partners together. There was this problem of branding and acknowledging each other's contribution. The coordination managed many partnership difficulties. We had to be supported by certain high-level organizations, such as the United Nations, which often helped the nation to put order in the various interventions. These are challenges that will have to be met in the long run.

In terms of collaboration with the authorities, we need to strengthen the structures that have been put in place because we realized that the authorities, at different levels, were not prepared to respond to epidemics. There were new officials who did not fully understand the role they had to play in their position. As a result, some of our actions in the different localities were slowed down. It took us some time to make them aware of their role in supporting the response, and to get them to adhere to the awareness messages. Often, when there was an event, everyone had an idea about it, which depended on their mood and emotion, an idea that was not based on factual information. So, they had problems harmonizing their ideas with those of the authorities, at all levels. These are concrete problems that we were encountering on the ground. There must be a certain harmony between the decision-makers, the administrative and political authorities, and the technical teams that have to give information to the authority in order to make decisions; not decisions that are taken "at the top", are imposed, and may prove to be unsuitable. These are the difficulties of the two lungs of management.

During Ebola, we had two types of diversity. There was a great diversity in international actors, about 53 of them who were not easy to coordinate on the ground. I would like to take this opportunity to invite all technical and financial partners, from the outset of an epidemic, to show respect for national directives, based on transparency, alignment, and accountability. Among national actors, there was a second diversity, not only with respect to returning nationals, but also with respect to NGOs and some national partners and local businesses.

One of the biggest challenges we encountered was with NGOs, the vast majority of which were involved in advocacy. We found that, in most cases, they did not master the awareness messages that were written by the coordination. Some of them gave contradictory messages regarding the transmission factors and knowledge of the disease. Some NGOs were much more concerned with their own business than with limiting the spread of the disease. Faced with this proliferation of NGOs, of which there were up to 400, we tried to establish four criteria for selection. The first criterion was to have an authorization or a decree for the creation of an NGO. The second criterion was that each NGO had to have a bank account. The third criterion was to have a headquarters. The fourth criterion, which eliminated many, was the presentation of a certificate of appreciation from a partner with whom the NGO had collaborated in the past. There was even a fifth criterion: that each NGO had to finance the communication plan it presented with 30% of its budget. In the end, of the 400 NGOs, only 10 met these criteria. We collaborated with the rest of these young people who helped us in this response. I will mention here the names of some of them. First, AGIL, with whom we collaborated in the area of sensitization. This NGO helped us particularly in Koropara. It facilitated the adhesion of the communities. There is also Tinkisso, which participated not only in sensitization, but also in the production of chlorine for spraying of contaminated areas. These are the two NGOs that stood out from the others. There were NGO associations made up of returning nationals, such as the nationals of Télémélé, famous for the control of the epidemic locally. And in Siguiri too, where the natives played a decisive role. In most of the prefectures where Ebola has occurred, returning nationals contributed a lot to fighting it. There have been youth associations that have been effective in helping us control the disease.

In terms of management, there has been strengths and weaknesses. A strength was that at the beginning, we all had the intuition that this was not a disease that was going to last and that we were going to control it with the support of the WHO and other partners. It is when the situation became obviously critical that we, with the national party, under the leadership of the Head of State, Professor Alpha Condé, launched an appeal to the nation and the international community to mobilize internal and external forces to eradicate the disease. Following this appeal, we received many responses among the institutions requested, both internally and externally. There were many volunteers, agents in Guinea who came forward to participate in this fight. Some companies also collaborated with us to help the State fight the disease. These were valuable contributions. Second, health workers mobilized with bravery to face this epidemic, despite the deaths recorded in our ranks. This did not disturb the staff or cause health workers to run away, to refuse to work or show reluctance. In fact, we had many more applicants than our needs required. Another strength was that we had the political commitment and unwavering support of the government, which was at the forefront of motivating us to address the health aspects. This support was there from the beginning. This is a summary of the different forces that Guinea was able to mobilize.

As for the weaknesses, we were quickly confronted with a lack of training, a lack of equipment, a lack of funding for this response, and a lack of infrastructure to accommodate the patients. These are the difficulties encountered at the beginning and which caused the delay in the treatment of many Guineans. That's why I said that as part of the preparation, this type of deficit must be corrected.

Among the prospects, we are pleased to have developed a plan to revive and strengthen our health system. We have set up the National Agency for Health Security (ANSS in French) to manage this type of epidemic or emergency. We are in the process of strengthening the financing of the response in the Republic of Guinea from partnership funds and funds from the national development budget. Since then, the budget allocated to the response and surveillance has increased, not only on the part of the State, but also on the part of partners, so that the agency is now well staffed and functioning. It is assisted in a punctual way in the different operations to enable it to face crises. All the areas I have just mentioned that were in short supply have seen remarkable improvements. Today, we have more than 38 treatment structures, whose capacities have been improved. At the beginning of this COVID-19 pandemic, we had only 500 or so beds available for treatment. As I write this, we have more than 1800 beds. So, that capacity has been greatly improved, to accommodate the many cases of COVID-19. In all areas, there has been a strengthening of capacity in terms of infrastructure, equipment, laboratories, human resources training, etc. Our logistical means have been strengthened.

This perspective must continue because we never know what the future and what the demands will be. We have a minimal capacity, and we must continue to strengthen it to improve its quality, to prepare for new events that may cause many victims.

Having lived through Ebola and managed it for two and a half years has allowed us to learn lessons and begin to build capacity. The first success, seen with COVID-19, is that we were able to diagnose the disease quickly. Instead of taking three and a half months, as it did during Ebola, when COVID-19 came along in March, we already had the equipment to detect it. The first case was detected in less than 48 hours. We already had the appropriate treatment and isolation centers. So, we immediately isolated the patients. This is the second achievement. As a third achievement, we already knew how to develop preparedness and response plans. Even before the first case was diagnosed, as soon as we learned that the disease was occurring, as soon as the WHO informed us, we developed a preparedness and response plan. We identified the prefectures at risk and the preparedness plan was based on the ten prefectures of Lower Guinea that were connected to the outside world by boats and planes. The first case arrived by plane. The plan was put into action as soon as the first case was detected. We quickly prepared equipment, reagents, supplies, treatment protocols, and all drugs were in place before the first case occurred. We quickly "recycled" the people who helped us during the Ebola epidemic to take care of patients. In terms of investigation, we also had prefectural teams already trained for this purpose. These teams launched investigations to identify contacts and place them under surveillance. We already had experience that prepared us to deal with COVID-19. With the lessons we learned, we quickly involved the communities. We launched the "Stop COVID-19 in 60 days, let's mobilize" strategy. Like "Zero Ebola in 60 days," this strategy helped us stop the spread of COVID-19. In short, we adapted our Ebola experience to begin the response to the COVID-19 epidemic.

We heard again some "Ebola readings". Some have claimed that it is a punishment from God. In the face of punishment, they say, no health remedy can work. According to them, it is because of our sins that God has punished us. This false belief shows that in the face of every event, one must take into account the interpretation of the community. This is the role of the Red Cross and the health services. We must not trivialize the community's interpretation but take the time to deconstruct it with factual and convincing arguments in order to gain their support and better implement strategies. From now on, we will have to take the time to understand all these interpretations, which vary from one place to another, and to prepare deconstruction messages, telling the population the truth about the event, to reassure them and ensure their collaboration. We had a hard enough time getting some of the traditional healers to understand that the "medicine" they had offered was not good. Unfortunately, people died while taking these fake remedies. We also had a hard time convincing some imams who believed that epidemics were the result of a curse from God and that their talisman could cure the disease. Unfortunately, we lost about ten imams (marabouts) who died during the Ebola epidemic. All these examples allowed us to demonstrate to their followers that this disease has an "objective" origin and that they must adhere to our response strategies.

Honours and Awards

Throughout my career I have received a few honorific distinctions and awards.

I obtained my first distinction in 1973, graduating with distinction for my baccalaureate, which exempted me from the university entrance exam.

The second one was obtained in 1980 at the Faculty of Medical Science in Havana, Cuba, where I was designated as the best foreign student at the end of my university studies, as reported by the newspaper Gramma on August 29th, 1980.

During Ebola, a third distinction was awarded to me by the French government through the Legion of Honor, which was given to me on July 14, 2015, during the French national holiday, at the French embassy in Guinea, in the presence of my wife and my son. It was a time of joy and encouragement for the efforts made in the fight against the Ebola virus disease. I kept this distinction and as the fight against Ebola was not over, I told myself that I would only wear this crown when the end of the Ebola epidemic in Guinea was declared. I thank the French government for this recognition which motivated me to continue to serve my country even more.

A fourth award was given to me by CDC during my visit in 2016, when I had the honor to visit this great country, the United States of America, which had provided a lot of support to the response. It was a unique opportunity: going to see how they work in their homeland was a very special experience for me. I was invited with my wife for a two-week stay in Atlanta and Washington. In Atlanta, I visited the CDC headquarters and talked with my friend, the then CDC Director, Tom Frieden, who spoke very highly of me during his trips to Guinea during the epidemic. We had fruitful discussions and I saw how he organized himself. The CDC offered me two things on that visit.

First, CDC offered a training of Guineans in field epidemiology, called the Field Epidemiology Training Program (FETP), which would enable Guineans to investigate and identify outbreaks in real time.

Second, it offered to strengthen the training and management of emergency operation centers to better coordinate interventions and their follow-up.

These trainings were funded by the CDC and are now paying off. Since 2017, we have had our own FETP program. In-country, we offer the three-month frontline level and the nine-month intermediate level. We also send Guineans to Burkina Faso to participate in the two-year advanced program. Between 2017 and September 2020, 179 Guineans completed the frontline training, 16 the intermediate level, and 11 the advanced level. We are proud that in such a short period of time, we have managed to have FETP graduates in all prefectures, all regions, and at the national level who are responsible for field investigations, but also surveillance data for diseases with epidemic potential. These agents have really transformed our capacity and have subsequently played a key role in the responses to the polio, measles and COVID-19 epidemics.

These trainings continue today, and we hope to make them an ongoing activity of the Ministry of Health to continue to improve our country's ability to identify and respond to outbreaks.

The concept of Emergency Operations Centers (EOCs) was new to our agency. CDC and its collaborators at Public Health Canada introduced it to us during Ebola. At that time, both agencies had created a center at the national level to improve communication and coordination between our coordination cell and all national and international partners. We were able to develop an EOC in each of the country's prefectures and each of Conakry's communes. Strategically, these EOCs are located in the Prefectoral and communal health departments (DPSs and DCSs) and continue, to this day, to accompany us in the management of epidemics and their data.

It was after that meeting that Tom Frieden surprised me at a conference with this award. He said, referring to me, that he was giving this high award to a contemporary epidemiologist in Africa who had proven himself in the response to Ebola in Guinea. It was very moving for me, the number of people who came to attend the event gave me comfort in my attitude to fight for my country, and why not for the international community, in the management of a pandemic.

I would like to pay special tribute to my friend and collaborator, the CDC Director in Guinea, Dr. Lise Martel. She hosted my wife and I in Atlanta in keeping with our Guinean customs of hospitality. I was able to eat foods that I had never eaten before, like pears, which I now eat here in Guinea. We visited touristic sites such as the Atlanta Aquarium, but also a fish farm where I was able to see the American way of growing fish, which I used to conceptualize my own project to alleviate the nutritional problems of my village.

The fifth distinction was the awarding of a certificate from Guinean nationals residing in Canada, which was also very moving. It took place at the Guinean Embassy in Ottawa, in the presence of Ambassador Saramady Touré, whom I have known for a long time. There I learned that the epidemic was also having an impact on Guinean nationals in Canada in the form of stigma. I realized that Guinean nationals continue to follow Guinean executives from outside the country. They follow them in their efforts to overcome diseases, but also for the development of our country, in general. This testimony was comforting for me because this recognition of our diaspora was present in Canada, as well as in France. This has comforted me and given me a patriotic spirit, coupled with the desire to continue to dedicate my life to the development of our country and the safeguarding of the health of our people.

A sixth award was given to me by the WHO following my management, participation and contribution to the implementation of the Merck vaccine trial. The WHO awarded me this honorary distinction of high significance, in my opinion, after validation by the *Lancet,* a reputable journal, in recognition of my contribution to the trial of this vaccine.

A seventh award was given to me by the President of the Public Health Agency of Canada during my visit in recognition of my *leadership* during the Ebola response. My visits to Quebec City, Montreal, and Ottawa allowed me to discuss the decentralization of the health system in Canada and the concept of incident management. I was able to visit emergency operation centers. I came back from these meetings with many documents.

In addition to these distinctions that I received from international institutions and Guinean nationals during my travels and visits after the victory against Ebola, I received many other satisfactions from associations and the Guinean civil society. National organizations have expressed their satisfaction with my commitment to this fight. I thank them from the bottom of my heart for this recognition.

The Head of State decorated Maggaret Thiam, the Director General of the WHO at this time with an honorary distinction for the success of the vaccination that stopped the Ebola epidemic in Guinea.

Testimonies about Dr. Sakoba Keïta

Professor René Migliani

Presentation by Professor René Migliani

Retired senior service physician from the Army Medical Corps as of May 1, 2014, born March 2, 1954 in Casablanca, Morocco.

Associate Professor at the Val-de-Grâce school, former holder of the Chair of Epidemiology and Prevention applied to the Armed Forces and former Director of the Centre for Epidemiology and Public Health of the Armed Forces. Specialist and teacher of public health with a focus on epidemiology and clinical research applied to the prevention of communicable diseases.

Professor René Migliani's contribution to the fight against Ebola in Guinea

Advisor, as part of the *"Task Force"* of the Ministry of Foreign Affairs of the French Republic, on the proposal of the Armed Forces Health Service, to the national coordinator of the fight against Ebola in Guinea, Dr. Sakoba Keita, and to the French Ambassador to Guinea, Bertrand Cochery, from October 12, 2014 to June 30, 2015.

During my stay in Guinea, consulting activities constituted the majority of my full-time activities with participation, alongside the coordinator, in all the daily technical and information meetings of the national coordination in the capital and in information, control strategy implementation and supervision missions in the field, as well as meetings led by the President of the Republic of Guinea, inter-ministerial meetings of the Prime Minister's Office, meetings of the Ministry of Health, and meetings with national and international technical and financial partners, including the World Health Organization, the

European Union, and other major United Nations organizations (UNICEF, World Food Programme). Each week, information on the evolution of the epidemic and the control measures implemented were presented during the conference organized at the Press House in the capital. Thus, for the press conference of the week of my arrival, my first advice to the coordinator was to provide the local media with the number of healed subjects in addition to the number of cases and deaths, in order to bring hope to the population. This indicator was subsequently included in all weekly press releases.

Among all the activities carried out during my stay, I set up in two weeks, with funding from France and with the help of a section of the French Civil Security and the French Armed Forces Health Service, the Ebola Caregivers Training Center (CFSE in French), located on the site of the military school in Manéah. This center allowed the training, from November 14, 2014 to March 31, 2015, of seven Guinean instructors, six trainers from the Guinean armed forces health service, and 257 trainees from twenty prefectures (doctors, nurses, hygienists, samplers and clinical research monitors).

In order to present the situation of the epidemic in Guinea and at the international level, I wrote an electronic bulletin every week from October 2014 to June 2015 in Guinea and then in France from July to December 2015, then a monthly bulletin from January to September 2016. Over time, this newsletter was sent to approximately 200 Guinean, and French and international partners. This information activity was complemented by the realization of information sessions for expatriates and French partners in Guinea.

To complete these activities, I participated in several conferences in Guinea, Dakar and France on the Ebola epidemic, in university training on Ebola in France and abroad after my stay in Guinea. Finally, I have written several scientific articles on the Ebola epidemic in Guinea.

France's main contributions to the fight against Ebola in Guinea

France has mobilized 110 million euros for action in West Africa, mainly for Guinea, with the reinforcement or construction of four Ebola treatment centers (ETCs), the construction by the French Ministry of Defense of a treatment center for caregivers (CTS) in Conakry, the dispatch of more than 200 health professionals to Guinea, and the financing of several clinical research studies. The French Embassy in Guinea has rehabilitated several airport runways in the interior of the country for the logistical activities of the fight.

Dr. Sakoba Keita, National Coordinator of the fight against Ebola in Guinea

During these nine months in Guinea, our collaboration was immediate, complete and trusting. I was able to measure how tirelessly Dr. Sakoba Keita worked, sparing neither time nor effort, without a moment of rest, to fight this epidemic. This was undoubtedly the most difficult of the twenty or so epidemics that he had to face throughout his career in the positions of responsibility that he held at the Ministry of Health. As national coordinator, he reported orally twice a day in detail to the President of the Republic, under whose direct authority he was placed since September 2014, after the reorganization of the fight. His willfulness, hard work, self-sacrificing qualities, mastery of the art of oratory, perfect knowledge of his country's health system, public health methods, and vast experience had undoubtedly been decisive in his successful appointment as national coordinator for the fight against Ebola. I had the honor to be his advisor. I learned from him. All those hours of work spent face to face, meals together, countless meetings and field missions have built a mutual respect and gradually, a sincere friendship.

Before the end of the Ebola epidemic, Dr. Sakoba Keita did not wait to project himself into the future by organizing Guinea's health surveillance. He was naturally appointed director of the new National Health Security Agency (ANSS in French) in 2016. This new establishment for the management and control of epidemics has demonstrated its interest and effectiveness in the fight against the COVID-19 pandemic, since March 2020.

Dr. Facinet YATTARA

I am Dr. Facinet Yattara, a public health physician, National Director of Community Health and Traditional Medicine at the Ministry of Health. I know Dr. Sakoba Keïta well. He is a manager of public health services. He has a lot of experience in managing epidemics because he was the head of the prevention division at the national directorate of prevention and community health at the Ministry of Health. He was one of the division heads of that directorate where I am now. The directorate had three divisions. The prevention division, the public health division, and the traditional medicine division. He was the division head of the national directorate of prevention and community health which is now the national directorate of community health and traditional medicine. In this capacity, he was responsible for the management of epidemics when Ebola occurred. Given his experience in this area, having managed several epidemics such as cholera, yellow fever, lassa fever, he was appointed to manage Ebola. After my years of service as an international civil servant, when I retired, I returned home to Guinea. I was doing independent consulting, both nationally and internationally. It was at this time that the Ebola epidemic occurred. I saw Dr. Sakoba regularly at work. He was on the radio, on television, every night, to explain the Ebola situation. It is important to remember that I have a lot of experience in managing epidemic and disaster situations, both in Guinea and elsewhere, because I have managed epidemics in other countries, such as the Democratic Republic of Congo (DRC). I managed the UNICEF health program there from 2001 to 2003, during the rebellion, when the country was divided in two; one part was under the leadership of the rebellion that did not want to hear anything related to the government, so the whole health system of that part was handed over to the United Nations and it was at that time that I was called to manage the UNICEF program in Eastern DRC, in Goma to be precise, for three years. During this time, there was not only this rebellion issue, but also the occurrence of epidemics, which are recurrent in the DRC. When I came back, I saw that Dr. Sakoba needed support. I called him to say that I had seen him on TV the day before and wanted to join him in the fight against Ebola. He asked me, “Do you want to help me ?”. I said yes. He said, "If you want to help me, I will send you to the part of the country that is causing me the most problems. He was talking about Macenta. At the time, it was the most epidemic area in Guinea. Macenta alone had 714 cases of Ebola, including 501 deaths; nearly 80% of the patients had died there. He created the position of prefectural coordinator in Macenta and assigned it to me. But what I remember about him is that first of all, by sending me there, he had confidence in me. It is true that there were national strategies, but there were necessary adaptations in the field and to put them into practice, one had to have previously worked in similar conditions. I think that's what helped us in Macenta. I only worked there for six months. During those months, we were able to control the disease. It was during this time that the epidemic moved to the Lower Coast, having started in the forest. As we gained ground on the disease in the forest, it moved to the Lower Coast, especially to Forécariah, Boffa and Dubreka. Especially Forécariah and Boffa. He asked me to come and help him in Boffa too. When we were finishing in Boffa, the disease exploded in Kamsar. This is where the situation was going to be critical for the country because of the CBG, the only factory that had not closed at the time. People were ready to close. So, when there was this explosion in Kamsar, he asked me to help him there too, which I accepted.

Towards the end of the epidemic in Boké, I told him: “I am leaving. I have helped the country so far”. He answered: "No, you can't leave. I still need you”. And that was another vote of confidence. He let all the other coordinators go and kept me. He told me that he wanted to restructure his surveillance system because during Ebola there was a failure of the surveillance system. He put me in charge of the surveillance department, which was not a surveillance department at the time. It was called a unit because the National Health Security Agency (ANSS) had not yet been created. It was called the National Ebola Coordination. That's how the surveillance unit was assigned to me.

Together, we restructured the surveillance system while setting up the most reliable part of the surveillance, which was the community level. After the surveillance system was in place, we began to cascade training from the central level to the field to have a surveillance system that could be resilient and effective in managing epidemics. Thus, the national coordination disappeared and gave way to the National Health Security Agency. The surveillance unit became the “integrated surveillance and response” department. I managed this department within the ANSS. All this happened because he trusted me since the time of Ebola. He understood that it was really necessary to continue with me to establish a surveillance system in the country that can manage epidemics. Today, the management of COVID-19 is better organized than it was during Ebola. It is because of the lessons learned from the Ebola epidemic that we have achieved this result. That is my first takeaway from him. He had confidence in me and gave me the latitude to make adaptations to national strategies on the ground. I have undertaken a lot of strategy changes based on the locality and context for the services. For me, that's important to note.

I think it was primarily his communication skills, his ability to work with people based on their experience, that made him better at managing the Ebola epidemic. He did not want to impose his wishes on us. I salute his ability to adapt and his capacity to mobilize partners and bring them together around a single fight. It is thanks to all his assets that he succeeded in managing this disease.

My final word is that I am very pleased with everything that we have been able to put in place through Sakoba's leadership in managing Ebola. I'm very pleased with what we've been able to give to the health system in terms of capacity to manage and respond to future epidemics. To me, that's important. If the health system is efficient and effective, that is the best thing for a country. We have restructured the surveillance system, but also the health system in general, by giving the health districts the capacity to monitor and respond to epidemics. Today, this is what is being used in the fight against COVID-19.

If you look on the internet, you can see that the health districts that have been affected by COVID-19 follow the same pattern in describing problems and sharing information on a daily basis. Every day, districts tell us about their different problems and projects. That is because of the capacity we gave them after Ebola. It is thanks to the setting up of this national coordination headed by Sakoba, who was really at the forefront of Ebola management.

Alhousseiny Makanera KAKÉ

I am a deputy in the National Assembly, president of the communication and new information technologies commission. I was Minister in charge of Communication at the time of the outbreak of Ebola in Guinea.

Ebola was a new disease in Guinea, so it was not well known. The first information we learned about it was that there were no drugs to treat it. As Minister of Communication at the time, we needed to gather a lot of information about the disease to better communicate about it. I called on the Ministry of Health and the Ministry of Communication, in the conference room of the Ministry of Communication, where we held a press conference with Dr. Sakoba Keïta, at the time, Director of Prevention.

He informed us that the virus had neither feet nor wings to spread and that man was the only means for its propagation. Thus, to cut the chain of transmission, I put to contribution the Ministry of Communication, passing by the religious leaders, the media and all the other ways and means which could allow that the good information is conveyed.

In all humility, the contribution of the Ministries of Communication and Health was decisive in driving out of Guinea this Ebola disease that struck us over 300 kilometers, from N'zerekoré to Forécareah; otherwise, we might have experienced the hecatomb. It took the political will of the government and the determination of experienced cadres, many of whom lost their lives, and others who came to take up the torch. Do you remember the drama of Womé where we lost eight people in one day? In spite of all this, they made an extraordinary sacrifice that allowed us to curb the disease.

First of all, it must be recognized that if Dr. Sakoba was coordinator of the response against this disease, it is because he deserved it, because there was, of course, another person in charge before him. If we unanimously decided that he should be promoted to this position, it is because, quite simply, he had irreproachable professional and human skills; in addition to that, he was devoted.

I would really like to commend this initiative because it has allowed us to gather a lot of necessary information that can be used as an effective means to put any other disease of the stature of Ebola out of action. I would like to take this opportunity to thank all those who have fought so hard to defeat the Ebola virus, especially Dr. Sakoba, who deserves our thanks.

Colonel Mamadou Saliou BALDÉ

I am the director of strategic studies for the National Gendarmerie High Command. At the time of the Ebola outbreak in 2014, I was designated to represent the Department of Defense and Security at the National Ebola Outbreak Coordination.

My mission was to ensure the defense and security of health care personnel and their equipment, since there was a strong reluctance on the part of the population in certain localities of Guinea where these health care personnel were lynched, others were even killed while on duty. I am thinking of the tragedy in Womé, and other incidents in Macenta, Guéckédou, Kissidougou...

I had heard about Dr. Sakoba Keita from the time he was managing cholera, but I only met him when I was assigned to him in 2014, as part of the fight against Ebola. What I remember about him is that he had a very buoyant *leadership*, because with all the controversies that marred the Ebola epidemic, his management was not at all easy. In spite of that, he managed flawlessly, first his team and then the pandemic. He is a personality of high standing, of impeccable competence in the field. He is an executive with an international dimension, if I may say so.

Dr. Momo CAMARA

I am a public health doctor, former secretary general of the Ministry of Health, but before this position, I had to assume other functions, notably the regional health inspectorate, the prefectural health directorate, and then I carried out the largest health project at the time, called the Bamako initiative.

At the time of the Ebola pandemic, on the instruction of Dr. Sakoba, I was in charge of coordinating the pandemic in the prefecture of Siguiri. In three months, we were at the tailing end in Siguiri, and he called me back for the same functions in the Conakry region and also to ensure the inspection of the Forécareah prefecture.

During the fight, I was in charge of coordinating all activities related to the fight against the epidemic in the Siguiri prefecture. In this sense, I was supposed to call all the stakeholders and make sure the activities were working well, according to the procedures, and that the resources made available to us were managed efficiently, so that the results would come quickly. After three months, we were able to put an end to Ebola in the Siguiri prefecture, thanks to the dedication of the entire team.

Dr. Sakoba Keïta is a brother, a friend of promotion, since we all studied in Havana for seven years in a certain rigor and since then, we have maintained very good relations. Humanly, he has supported me a lot. We worked together and we were able to propose an idea that changed the functioning of our health system, when I was then Secretary General of the Ministry of Health. This idea consisted in preparing a succession by preparing our medical colleagues who were in charge of disease surveillance and today, this has revolutionized our health system.

I remember Dr. Sakoba as a man of integrity, dedication and team spirit. He is a *leader* who has always been able to achieve the goals he sets for himself.

To write a testimony on our journey is salutary, I find, because in Guinea, it is not everyone who can write. However, we do very beautiful things that deserve to remain in posterity; it could be a stimulant for the young generation. On that note, I simply take my hat off to him.

Colonel Rémy LAMAH

As a physician by profession, I was Minister of Health at the time of the Ebola epidemic in Guinea. As soon as we were informed of the outbreak of the Ebola virus in southern Guinea, we contacted Dr. Sakoba Keita who was, at the time, the head of the division in charge the epidemics. He automatically sent a team of experts, led by Dr. Lamine Koïvogui, to Guéckédou and Macenta to take a first sample, which was sent to France for testing.

Meanwhile, I was on a mission to Yomou. It was on the way that I was contacted by the Minister of State, Chief of Staff of the Presidency, Dr. Diané. From there, I turned around and went back to Conakry to read the declaration of the Ebola epidemic.

The next day, I went to meet Dr. Sakoba in his office in Kaloum. He gave me the first tools to fight the disease that I had to transport to the affected localities, and then continue my journey to N'Zerekore to complete the mission that the President had entrusted to me. During this time, I must admit that I was very much solicited by my counterparts, the Ministers of Health of the sub-region, who were wondering how to prevent the pandemic, since it was completely new and caused great fear.

Dr. Sakoba Keïta being very experienced, in collaboration with the government, took all the necessary measures to contain the disease in the first affected localities, so that it would not spread. The adventure was not a rosy one, taking into account the ups and downs that marred the course of our struggle. For example, the dramatic event in Womé where we lost eight cadres treated in a dehumanizing way, and the difficulties related to burials because in Africa, there are many ceremonies related to burial. Wanting to change this practice could not but arouse indignation in the population. Yet it was vital.

I must admit that Dr. Sakoba Keïta is of unprecedented efficiency, irreproachable courage and, above all, driven by a love of work, because I assure you that during the entire time of the response, he had absolutely no rest. He is also a great technician; it must be emphasized. When it was decided to set up a coordination committee through which everything would be coordinated for the response, in the presence of a UN representative, people immediately rushed to take the lead in the coordination, believing that they could benefit from everything that could be done. In spite of these negotiations, Dr. Sakoba Keita, because of his devotion and self-sacrifice, was unanimously the ideal choice and the President of the Republic. Professor Alpha Conde was quick to confirm his appointment as coordinator. Dr. Sékou Condé, who is his friend, with whom, moreover, he studied medicine in Cuba, was his deputy. Thus, the response team was well prepared to live up to expectations.

It was a comforting feeling for me to make my modest contribution as Minister of Health at such a critical time in our history. The management of Ebola has been a rich experience for me as a military doctor. The Ebola virus also allowed Guinea to strengthen its health system. It was an exhilarating moment. With the courage of the entire corporation, we can only congratulate ourselves on the work that was done.

Fodé Tass SYLLA

I am the general manager of the national television, a journalist and historian.

At the formation of the coordinating committee for the fight against the Ebola epidemic, my Minister of Communication and Information at the time, Alhousseny Makanera Kaké, sent me to represent him at the session of the inter-ministerial committee that was to deal with the disease. It was there that I made contact with Dr. Sakoba Keïta, Dr. Sékou Condé and their team. Thus, I was asked to lead the communication around the disease during the whole response.

As the communication officer for the Ebola epidemic coordination, my role was to ensure the design and dissemination of all awareness messages that came from the different international organizations, with UNICEF as the main partner.

Concerning Dr. Sakoba Keïta, despite his sometimes-volcanic character, I don't think there are two people in Guinea who could handle health issues like Ebola so well at the time. The day the WHO wanted to set up the committee to fight the epidemic, I was with Dr. Sakoba and Colonel Rémy Lamah, Minister of Health. We were the only three Guineans to attend the session that was held in Accra, Ghana.

We became almost twins throughout the process. Some people gave me the sobriquet of chief of workers at the time of the installation of the cell of the national coordination of the fight against Ebola in Kaloum, which later became the ANSS, a way to perpetuate the achievements of the fight against Ebola.

Basically, we can say that Sakoba is very efficient, courageous and especially committed to serve his nation.

I don't think it is necessary to give any advice to young doctors to adopt Dr. Sakoba's example. Everyone who saw him work during Ebola knows that he is a reference. In fact, for us who led the coordination, at the time, everyone was a reference in his field. For example, I was in communications, Colonel Baldé in security, Konaté, from the central pharmacy, in logistics ... and so many others.

Apart from the indoctrination of the population by political opponents, who made them believe that the disease was imported by the President, the biggest obstacle was the circulation of rumors. We had to deconstruct them in a rational way, with clear, factual arguments. We are proud of the work we did because the response system we left in place after Ebola, I don't think exists in any other country. The proof is that since the announcement of the COVID-19 pandemic that is ravaging the world, Guinea has not even recorded one hundred deaths. This shows the reliability of the means we have to fight against possible epidemic diseases.

I was very happy to serve my country during Ebola. It has been a very rewarding adventure for me, as I have been able to gain insight into the medical world through my various contacts with doctors all over the world, and if needed, I will be able to share these experiences.

TRAORÉ Youssouf

I am Traoré Youssouf, president of the Guinean Red Cross. I was a member of the national coordination of the fight against the Ebola epidemic, head of the unit of centralization and management of bodies during the response against this epidemic in Guinea.

My team and I took care of the safe and dignified burial of the bodies, as well as the transfer of the patients to treatment centers due to the lack of centers in certain regions or to the saturation of certain centers. Under instruction from the national coordinator, Dr. Sakoba Keita, we assumed other functions, such as the collection of samples from red zones or active foci, which was assigned to us after we received appropriate training.

Dr. Sakoba is a specialist in public health, who has a perfect command of the medical field. Moreover, he has shown impeccable courage by always remaining lucid at the front, despite the enormous difficulties encountered throughout the process. He has been able to assume his responsibility with accuracy and thanks to his good management, our country has benefited from great attention from donors and international institutions, which have provided a significant amount of material support to Guinea.

At the end of the health crisis, the Ebola epidemic made our health system competitive in the sense that our doctors benefited from a lot of experience. Treatment centers have sprung up all over the regions of Guinea, which has enabled us to better contain this COVID-19 pandemic, compared to other countries where it is causing enormous damage.

Finally, I really liked the idea of working with Dr. Sakoba Keïta, who is a leader who listens to everyone. He is the one who called on me, again, when the COVID-19 pandemic broke out, to lead this new adventure together again. We were both victims of this coronavirus and admitted to the Centre for Epidemiological Treatment (CT-Epi). That's how much we are exposed by being on the front line.

Dr. Pepe BILIVOGUI

I am Dr. Pépé Bilivogui, public health physician. Currently at the Ministry of Health, without a position for the moment. During the Ebola epidemic in our country, I led a number of activities with Dr. Sakoba Keïta. When the epidemic was declared, I was identified as the first operational coordinator based in the Forest region and more specifically in the epicenter, i.e., Guéckédou. I was working on the coordination of stakeholders because there were many partners. They needed an executive at the central level, and I was the national director of public health. So, I was identified by the department to go and do that job. That was the first job I took on, coordinating all the activities. This consisted of the operational identification of activities to stop the epidemic.

Every morning, we met with all the partners to plan the activities together. The achievements were monitored in the field, and then we came to do the evaluation at the base.

Everything we needed for the fight was identified in a plan that we called "emergency response plan".

The execution of this plan allowed us to identify the useful means and resources, all that was necessary for the implementation of the management, the follow-up of contacts, but above all the surveillance, the evolution of the disease, the management of the patients, that is to say how things should be organized with the diagnoses, the identification of suspected cases, and laboratory confirmation. We conducted this whole series of activities together, with all the partners, and the national part.

The epidemic lasted three years in its entirety since it really started in December 2013. For the Guéckédou mission, I spent six months in the field. I only came back once to see my family in Conakry.

I am unable to admit who scouted me for this mission, because Dr. Sakoba called me and said, “Did you get your mission order ?” I asked, “What mission order?” He said, surprised, “Didn't anyone inform you ?” I answered “no” and it was he who told me that I had to go to Guéckédou for the mission I mentioned above. I went to see Dr. Sakoba, and he explained the details of my mission. I said "ok" because it was Dr. Sakoba who had called me.

When I went on mission to Guéckédou, I was in communication with the central level. The transmission of information between the central level and the operational level was done by me, and the setting up of all the so-called databases was under my authority, with the partners.

Thank God, I already had some experience in the field since I managed many epidemics when I was prefectural director of health, in particular cholera for seven years in Boké. Then, during the same period, I managed a yellow fever epidemic. There are many similarities between the management of yellow fever and Ebola. Even apart from that, I had a lot of other experience in managing epidemics. Dr.

Sakoba knew why he had chosen me, and he appreciated my field operations, as did the minister. At the time, it was Colonel Remy Lamah, the medical officer.

With Dr. Sakoba, we were on the ground. After we beat the epidemic, I was promoted to the national Ebola coordination as head of the epidemiological surveillance unit. It was all about surveillance, in collaboration with our partners. This time, Dr. Sakoba was the coordinator of the national Ebola coordination unit. There were many partners, including Doctors Without Borders, the World Health Organization, UNFPA, which is now called UNFPA, UNICEF, the Guinean Red Cross, and the International Federation of Red Cross and Red Crescent Societies, among others, who were able to intervene in this process.

Dr. Sakoba was the coordinator of the national Ebola cell. I knew him well before that and knew that he had experience in fighting epidemics. I also knew that he was a well-trained executive with a lot of experience. In short, he was up to the task. Our collaboration was very fruitful. I represented him everywhere, with the government and outside, because Dr. Sakoba was so busy that he could not go away. I also had the opportunity to be his substitute during his leaves, I was the one who coordinated. We worked closely together. Afterwards, I became his advisor, in charge of the mission.

Concerning what we can remember about him, I have already mentioned his competence in the technical field, and this is the most important, at least in terms of epidemic management. Dr. Sakoba has had a good career, he has benefited from it. He really has a proven technical competence. He is a reference, not only in Guinea, but also, I dare to say, in Africa, and why not worldwide? Because we have seen him at work and personally, I have appreciated his abilities. He works very, very hard. He has a clear patriotic conscience. I'm not throwing flowers at him, I'm describing what he really is, from my perception. Whenever I have worked with him, there has always been a good relationship between us. Dr. Sakoba is a seasoned professional, with all his experience, his intellectual capacity, and his undeniable work conscience. He works tirelessly. We were together sometimes until 7 or 8 pm and we left the office together. We would come back at about 7 or 8 in the morning. In spite of his health problem, he held on for his country. He gave the best of himself; he gave his body and soul.

Dr. Sakoba knew how to manage everyone, he gave himself in his mission to fight against this epidemic and despite the workload, he always remained very good with his collaborators, respectful.

Personally, I am available because, when there was a reshuffle in the Department of Health, they abolished the National Directorate of Hygiene that I headed. But I am proud of what I was able to do with Dr. Sakoba Keita and many other things in my career. Unfortunately, there has not yet been a decree since the last appointments. This decree which eliminated the national direction of hygiene did not take me into account. So, I am waiting for another assignment, and I am still a reserve officer, ready to intervene at any time, as it was the case for Ebola. The coronavirus outbreak is less dangerous than the Ebola outbreak. In terms of mortality, everyone understands that the difference between the two is obvious.

I thank Dr. Sakoba for his frank collaboration with me and I think he remains a reference. There are some people with whom the intensity of the activities made Dr. Sakoba angry, and the collaborators sometimes reproached him for being angry, but he was not mean and socially, I appreciate him. He has a sense of humor in everything he does. I found him to be professional, intellectually capable, and morally upright. His few moments of anger are understandable because he was under pressure. In spite of everything, he managed and was still able to face a second threat, which is a global pandemic. He is to be commended, thanked, and congratulated.

Dr. Sekou CONDÉ

I am Dr. Sekou Condé, currently Secretary General of the Ministry of Health.

In 2014, our country was facing a serious epidemic. Given the specifics related to the disease, it caused a lot of deaths. We had an extremely high mortality rate compared to COVID-19, as we lost almost 60% of infected patients, with all the consequences that this had, both on health professionals and in the general population. I remember as a sad memory the loss of 115 agents out of 212, who were infected. They died on the battlefield.

When I think of the epidemic, I think of the situation of these families, that there was no special honor. That is what I regret today. The steps have been taken for some time, but in our administration, there is no logic of continuity. Otherwise, the problem was raised at the highest level, instructions were given to take care of the families, and it was done, they received their pension. When a person dies while working, there are expenses related to the education of children and everything that follows. The pension does not provide for all these needs. Unfortunately, we receive calls from families who were affected. What I remember is that there are some who were murdered, it was not the disease that took them, they went for the awareness sessions and they were killed. When there are situations like that, I think that humanly and socially, what we should do is to think about these families, to provide reparations. It's like soldiers who have fallen on the battlefield.

The three most affected countries were Guinea, Sierra Leone, and Liberia, but we did not adopt the same strategies, we preferred the participatory approach. With the lessons learned, we managed better than the others. That is why, towards the end, countries came to learn from our experience. That is why, most recently, when there was the Ebola epidemic in the DRC, they asked for Guinean expertise.

When the disease began, I was the national director of health care institutions. Afterwards, I was asked to support the response. One of the important elements of the fight was the organization of treatment. This could not be achieved without seconding someone to do this. So, after much discussion, the position of deputy coordinator was created. I was not too "hot" to take up this position because I already had other duties, other obligations, but one fine day, I was surprised by the President of the Republic who announced to me: "Well, there is a decree that will come out today and you will join the position, there is no discussion". I went without discussion because for me it was a sign of confidence. When I came in, like all organizations, especially in an emergency situation, you had to avoid jurisdictional conflicts. You have to structure an organizational base because you can't do it in a mess. I spoke with Sakoba, who was a good collaborator, for a long time. I told him: "Given my administrative experience, we need to divide the tasks, you are the coordinator, and I am the deputy coordinator. In a response, there are functions. The coordination function, the administration function, the management function, the financial function, the logistical support function, and the external action function. You, by virtue of your position, are going to be dealing primarily with all the coordination, the meetings, and you're going to be supporting the oversight. Now, anything that is operational and is going to require a lot of administration, financial analysis, report writing, logistical support, human resources organization, I will take care of that. On this basis, we agreed and the first thing I did was to say that the administration would not work if there were no internal regulations. We developed a set of bylaws. Secondly, I had a procedure manual developed. This allowed everyone to do what they should do, especially in an emergency situation.

Afterwards, of course, with Ebola, we had to develop projects, because there were many partners who are at the service of development. The African Development Bank, the French Cooperation, the World Bank... With the institutions, it is necessary to develop specific projects, so I coordinated the development of projects. Then, I had to follow up on their execution, report monthly on training, because the money from the partners is subject to periodic audits. From a financial point of view, this is what I did. Then, I coordinated the operational activities, the human resources, how to recruit them, how to sign contracts and deploy staff in the field. The logistical means, how to distribute them and on what criteria, and then everything related to the operational environment of the response.

Dr. Sakoba is a friend I know well because we lived together. We both studied medicine as interns in Cuba and when we returned, we were both transferred to the interior of the country. He went to Siguiri, I went to Lola and after a while I went to France. When I returned, I was appointed director of healthcare institutions. He was then regional director of health in Mamou and Boké and when I arrived, we obviously needed a certain dynamic in the prevention division. We wrote a call for applications among the regional health directors. We organized it and he was the best placed because what is important is the performance of results. He came to prevention and that's where he was appointed coordinator from, so that means we know each other a little bit! He is a very committed person, sometimes even a little over-committed since he does not measure the consequences or the pitfalls. He is very open with his colleagues. He can be angry, but he is an excellent and competent manager, only what he doesn't know how to do, and this depends on his administrative culture, is to follow the procedure scrupulously. As a result, he is always in an emergency situation, he wants to reach his objectives quickly, forgetting the procedures, whereas when you forget the procedures, sometimes it catches up with you. He was very committed, that's why I said, at the beginning, that we had to divide the tasks. And it is rightly that he received the award of the French Republic: The Legion of Honor.

Lise Martel

I am the CDC country director in Guinea. I came to Guinea for Ebola. The outbreak was declared in March 2014 when the first cases in the forest area were detected. I arrived in Guinea in September 2014.

The CDC is the Center for Disease Control and Prevention. It is a United States federal agency responsible for the health of Americans.

We have offices in about sixty countries around the world, but Guinea was not one of them in 2014. When there are epidemics, outbreaks, something really worrisome, the CDC usually sends investigators to the field to assess the extent of the problem and see how to help. At the time, I was working in Côte d'Ivoire on Ebola epidemic preparedness. When the first cases of Ebola appeared in Conakry, I was asked: "You are not far away, you are in Côte d'Ivoire. Couldn't you go and tell us what is needed in Guinea for emergency management? Should we send people there?" When I got here, I told Atlanta "Send everything you have”. A lot of CDC people do not speak French. CDC Atlanta was able to send about 15 people to help lead the response here.

I was planning to go back to Côte d'Ivoire to continue my work there, but Côte d'Ivoire told me "No, you are in Guinea, so you can't come back here unless you do 90 days of quarantine.” They were afraid. I told Atlanta that Ivory Coast did not want me to go back, and they asked, "Can you stay in Guinea? "I gladly agreed. I stayed here to help with the response.

I went to the Pita building and that is where I met Dr. Sakoba. I wanted to do what I could to help. My specialty was emergency management. I wanted to help structure the response. Dr. Sakoba was in charge. I met with his secretary, Mrs. Sangaré, and sat down with my computer on the corner of her desk. After a few days, Dr. Sakoba asked me, "Do you want an office? "I refused, because I liked being there, I could see what was going on and what the needs were. For me, it was easier to help if I was close to him.

The first few weeks, Dr. Sakoba would call me "CDC". He would be in his office and he would yell, "CDC, come here! "And I would come to his office. He would ask me if I could help him with this or that. People would send him samples, so he would ask me: "Can you figure it out? Are these tests good? Are these medications good or not? I would say, "Yes, of course! " I did not know personally the answers, but the CDC is a 13,000-person organization that is divided into small, specialized areas. There are specialists for Ebola, specialists for coronavirus, specialists for just about every disease, laboratory specialists, etc. If I don't know, that is okay, I can contact the specialists in the field and ask them. That's how it works with the CDC. With us, it's not just the expertise of the person in the field that counts, but also the expertise of others at the agency that can help us, if we need it. As we have offices in about 60 countries around the world, working on research into diseases with epidemic potential, there is also a network in which we can go and find people to help us. For example, in this context, when we were looking for Ebola cases, we brought in colleagues from the DRC. They had gone through the kind of training we needed here, so we brought them in to help. There were people from all over. The world's leading Ebola expert came, someone who has organized a lot of responses, in DRC and in different countries, Pierre Rollin. He is retired now. At the time, Pierre Rollin was the great expert on all hemorrhagic fever diseases, including Ebola. Pierre was sent to the forest area of Guinea with the first CDC team, in March 2014. Pierre and his team worked in the Macenta and N'Zerekore area. It was not worrisome until the disease made its way to the capital. Then, we became very concerned. At first, the disease was only in small villages of the forest area where there are more contact between animals and humans. People who prepare bush meat, who go hunting were thought to be more likely to be in contact with the virus that was believed to come from bats or monkeys. Until then, it had not reached a large city. It was the first time in history that Ebola entered a major city, and it did in three countries, Guinea, Sierra Leone, and Liberia at the same time. It was pretty catastrophic.

Since September 2014, CDC has had a consistent presence in Guinea, and opened an office in September 2015. As the epidemic lasted, the CDC considered it best to open an office to have a stable presence on the ground, at least for the duration of the epidemic. Initially, the idea was that after the epidemic, the office would likely close. The epidemic lasted two years. CDC decided to stay another year "just in case"... Then there were a lot of problems with measles, and we stayed a little longer still. And then, when the coronavirus came along, it was decided that the office would stay open at least until September 2022.

Dr. Sakoba was one of the first people I worked with when I came here. Because there was no CDC office at the time, I was not the director then, I was just one of the CDC people who came to help.

I was impressed with Dr. Sakoba. He is smart and competent, and has a lot of field experience. He is also charismatic and able to make people work together. And that was specific to Guinea because in other countries, leadership was often assumed by international partners. Here, it was really Dr. Sakoba who was managing the epidemic and we, the partners, rallied behind him.

I was impressed with his wisdom. The international partners and many people would come and say, "Okay, doctor, we'll explain how you should proceed". I looked at him and thought: "He who has fought fourteen epidemics of cholera, yellow fever, meningitis and who knows Guinea from top to bottom, who is a doctor and an epidemiologist, who knows public health... What can these people tell him that he doesn't already know?" But he listened, he was polite, patient with all of them. I don't know how he did it, but that's a huge quality. Wisdom never left him. Sometimes, when some were a bit annoyed with partners, he would calm us down: "Wait, everyone can bring something. We'll work together".

He quickly gained the confidence of all the international partners. After that, it became easier because the money started coming in; so much money with Ebola that many did not know what to do with it. We had difficulty spending all that money. Dr. Sakoba knew what to do with it.

When the position of Director of CDC Guinea was created, a coworker recommended I apply. I spoke with Dr. Sakoba. He told me that it would be very good if I became director, we worked so well together.

I admire Dr. Sakoba as a professional, but also as a human being. He is one of the most patriotic people I know. Because of all his qualifications and qualities, with Ebola he is now recognized worldwide, including in the United States. You say "Dr. Sakoba", everyone knows who you are talking about. He is a reference in the epidemiological field and not only for Ebola, but also for cholera and several other epidemic-prone diseases. He also has a lot of experience with leprosy.

I admire the way he did everything he could for the good of his countrymen. It's amazing. I have a lot of respect for that. He is charismatic, he is humble. I have never seen him brag about anything, other people sing his praises.

With the epidemic, there was a lot of tension, a lot of politics behind the scenes. There were a lot of misunderstandings with all the different cultures and languages. The response was very complex to manage. I looked at him and wondered how a man of his age, in two years, didn't take a vacation. I think in two years he took one week off to go see his mother. It was pure dedication. He would have died before he stopped, and I thought if he was going to continue, I should continue too.

Ebola showed that Guinea could lead and manage a serious epidemic, with the help of others. All the lessons learned during Ebola have been well applied since. Now, when we look at how Guinea manages the coronavirus, it is so much better, thanks to the fruit of the experiences accumulated and to the vision of Dr. Sakoba. For example, people wanted to build temporary structures for treatment and Dr. Sakoba said: "You must build permanent structures, I don't want anything temporary". Treatment centers were built in each district and are now used for COVID-19. These are free-standing structure that ensures that the main hospital does not get infected by easily transmitted diseases such as tuberculosis, Ebola, and COVID-19. Highly contagious patients can be isolated in these separate structures that are still under the responsibility of the hospital with assigned doctors and nurses.

I also had the opportunity to get to know Dr. Sakoba more personally. Because he has done such outstanding work with Ebola, he received an award from the CDC in Atlanta. I traveled for two weeks with him and his wife, one in Washington and one in Atlanta. It was their first trip to the United States. So I heard many of his comments, and observed his open-mindedness. Every time he discovered something positive, he thought about how to adapt it to

Guinea issues and change his way of doing things to improve himself. Here are some small examples.

One day he said to me, "You know, Lise, CDC meetings never last more than an hour, most of the time are only 30 minutes. Meetings start and end on time. There is always an agenda and at the end of each meeting, there are action points. In Guinea, we don't do that. You have seen our meetings, they last two or three hours. We finish without action points, we don't know who is going to do what. When I go back to Guinea, we will do meetings your way". Back in Guinea, at the very first ANSS meeting, participants were excited and asked him, "So doctor, how was America?" His answer was: "I learned something in America, there people always start meetings on time. Now we'll do that here too." People laughed. He said, "Next Thursday, if you are not here on time, the door of the meeting room will be closed. You won't be able to get in." People laughed, once again. The following Thursday, he told his assistant, "In two minutes, as soon as it's time for the meeting, you're going to lock the door." Half the people were not there, they were banging on the door. Dr. Sakoba started the meeting and half an hour later, he looked at how much time was left and asked them to hurry up and discuss the action points. The following week, people were rushing to get there on time. Since then, these meetings start on time and end on time. He doesn't have three-hour meetings anymore, there are always concrete action items, things to check on, that were proposed the week before compared to what was actually done. People thought this could not be done because as a general rule, all meetings start late in Guinea...except with Dr. Sakoba. If he says it starts at 9:00, at 9:00 you better be there!

In Atlanta, when we were driving, he was looking around, curious about everything. At one point he said to me, "Lise, this morning to go to CDC, should we leave early? ». I was puzzled: "Why doctor? ». "Because it's raining. " I answered:

“It doesn't matter, it doesn't make any difference.” We left in the car and he was surprised: "Lise, it's raining but I don't see any water, where is the water? ». "Look at the roads doctor, they are designed in such a way that the water goes away on the sides, there are holes, sewers. It's connected underneath, there's no water accumulated on the roads. He looked and thought before starting a discussion about how Guinea could benefit from such a system. Guinea was always on his mind.

Another time, I asked him: "What do you want to eat?" He answered: "What I really want are fresh fruits and vegetables. I took him to Whole Food where you put what you want in a small container. It is weighed on a scale and the price is calculated by weight, no matter what you buy. I took him and his wife on a tour and he discovered a lot of produce that he didn't know about because you can find these types of fruits and vegetables in the United States but not in Guinea. His wife was looking for things she knew, she said, "That's chicken, okay, we'll take it.” Dr. Sakoba filled his plate with things he didn't know and sat down and tasted everything. I looked at him and wondered who else would do that. Most people seek the comfort of something they know, but he was always drawn to new experiences. He tasted pears and when he came back to Guinea, he told me, "Lise, did you know that I saw pears at the market? I asked Mrs. Sangaré to buy some for me.” I think this illustrates a childlike openness to discovering something new. It made my trip with him very interesting because he was open to learning, to experiencing something new all the time.

Dr. Sakoba has a good sense of humor, too. He always sees the humor in situations. Before he left, he said to me, "Lise, I need to talk to you. I know that in the United States, people drive too fast. Could you ask the driver not to drive too fast, I have a lot of trouble with that. More than 100 kilometers per hour is not good.” I answered: "Doctor, it won't be too difficult because I am your driver!” He laughed.

When we got there, I told him: "Doctor, you wait for me here with your luggage, I'll go get the vehicle and I'll come back". When I came back with the vehicle, he looked at me and laughed out loud. He explained: "You're our driver, really? I thought you were joking." It's a cultural difference because in the United States, people don't have a driver, they drive themselves. They also do their own cooking and cleaning. Dr. Sakoba is very introspective and thought often about the cultural differences. Back in Guinea, in a meeting, he said to the audience while talking about me: "You see Lise, she has a lot of respect for us Guineans, because when she is in Guinea, she doesn't dress like she does in the United States." He understood that for me, it is very important to be respectful. If I go to see the Grand Imam, I wear long sleeves, and my hair is covered. He understood that and it created a bond of mutual respect between us. I found that it gave us a lot of latitude in our relationship because when I made a mistake, I could go to him and say, "Dr. Sakoba, I made a mistake. He would say, "Okay, we'll fix it together," rather than getting angry and putting it in front of the partners; always in the spirit of fixing rather than blaming. I never saw him blame the partners.

Dr. Sakoba honored me by bringing me to his village, Sanankoro. I thought that the CDC office was closing for good, so I said: "Doctor Sakoba, I think this is the last year, the office will close". He said: "Lise, before you leave, I want to bring you to my village and introduce you to my mother. When he came to Canada, he also had met my mother. We went to his village where I met the elders. I didn't understand everything because people spoke in the local language. Suddenly, two goats were brought in and pictures were taken. My driver then asked me: "Madam, are you going to bring your goats back to Conakry?". I looked at him puzzled. He added: "They are your goats, they were given to you, don't you understand? It is not easy to fit two goats into a CDC vehicle on a mission! They also gave me fresh honey. Two friends from the United States were with me. The locals gave them traditional clothes. I told Dr. Sakoba that I could not see how to bring the goats back to Conakry. He said, "We can kill them and cut them into pieces. You can bring back the piece". I was truly touched that people give me two goats but ended up giving them to Dr. Sakoba's mother.

I was happy to see Dr. Sakoba's village. It is a modest place without much electricity, with a small generator that produced a little current, and three water pumps. Dr. Sakoba's residence there is also modest in infrastructure but rich in its people. He is surrounded by family there. I saw the love, the affection of his people. People came and teased him; children took him by the hand. He is a benefactor of his village, respected and loved. I looked at him and I was very touched. I thought that this was his nature. He is in his village as he was in the United States. He is the same person. I often ask him how his mother is doing, and he asks me about mine, because we have journeyed together. Wontanara.

Boubacar DIALLO

I am Boubacar Diallo, a Malian national and a public health physician. I arrived in Conakry on February 5, 2014 on behalf of the CDC in Atlanta. There was a joint program between the CDC and WHO in the framework of polio eradication, for which the CDC recruited me. I had two weeks of training in Atlanta, and then they sent me to Guinea, where I was based at the WHO office. I started working on measles and polio in February. Around March 21st, if I remember correctly, we were notified that there was an Ebola outbreak in Guéckédou, which was the epicenter, in the forest. Immediately, WHO mobilized and since Dr. Sakoba was the national director of the surveillance division, we gathered around him to work on a response plan.

As soon as Ebola started, the WHO office decided to stop all ongoing programs, and everyone was mobilized for this new epidemic. On March 26, I was deployed to Guéckédou, in the epicenter of the disease. So, I worked only four days with Dr. Sakoba in Conakry. From March 26 to September 10, 2014, I was based in the forest region.

I have worked in eight countries: Guinea, Nigeria, Canada, England, Madagascar, Niger, DRC and finally, Congo Brazzaville where I am currently based. I must admit that I have never seen a more social person than Dr. Sakoba. He is very human, very cooperative, and very concerned about the problems of people around him. He is humble and has a way of dealing easily with all his collaborators; that is on the social level. We have been so close, he and I, that we have finally been like brothers.

One day, my father was unwell, having a stroke, and there was no plane. I was given a WHO vehicle to drive. Sakoba was already in Kankan to supervise. He told me, "You will sleep at my place and tomorrow morning, very early, you will continue to the border." He waited for me; I was with my driver. I came, I ate, I exchanged with him and I fell asleep. At 5 o'clock in the morning, he woke me up. It was at his mother's house. Every time, he invites me to go and see his farm in the village, but I haven't had the time to do it yet. So he is a very social person.

Professionally, he is one of a kind. I have never seen anyone like him. I've worked in a lot of countries with the Ministry of Health and I've never seen anyone more professional than Sakoba. He is so honest, too. If we have succeeded in Guinea, it is because of him. Sakoba has a strong leadership, he is charismatic and that is his strength. He is very intelligent, when it comes to epidemics, there are no two like him in Africa.

Sakoba will say that he worked with everyone, but he was closest to me during the entire management of the epidemic, when I left Guéckédou, in September 2014, to be the WHO focal point for its coordination. I worked with him; I was the closest person to him. Our relationship was very open, we told each other everything and we moved forward. He trusted me because I studied in the United States, Canada, England, and I took epidemic courses, too. We complemented each other.

Whenever we were in trouble, I would go to his office and we would discuss strategies, just the two of us. All the strategies that were initiated and created were by Sakoba and me.

The first strategy was enhanced surveillance coupled with education. He said that and we wrote the project protocol.

His honesty has made all donors trust him. He doesn't like corruption and that is a strong point. That's why he is confident, he knows he is honest, he doesn't steal anyone's money and when he is given money, he uses it wisely. So, donors have trusted him and even I, as a partner, have mobilized a lot of funds for the country in the context of Ebola under the leadership of Dr Sakoba. At WHO, we are able to mobilize funds easily. We mobilized so much that after my mission, I left money behind at the office to continue to help his new structure. And all of this was made possible by his leadership, honesty and candor.

Also, he is very political; not in the classical sense, but in the professional sense, he knows how to manage partners, whenever there are conflicts. I was surprised that Sakoba did not become Minister of Health. Guinea will lose a lot. This man would have straightened out the Guinean health system. There is no African who knows the health system of a country better than Sakoba.

If it wasn't for Sakoba's leadership, we would never have ended this epidemic before 2017 in Guinea. I am aware of that. It would have been a sham. He had so many resources released! Imagine, we saw vehicles by the hundreds. We gave them to all the prefects, the DPS, the DCS and everywhere, we equipped them. I come from the DRC, after a year of fighting Ebola, I was coordinating the action at the WHO level, but you cannot compare the two responses and that is what I said every time. I said: "We must imitate Guinea Conakry". In DRC, it was going in all directions and they could not benefit from much money because there was not a good transparency in the management. So Sakoba, for me, is really unique and Guinea has an asset in his person, it must exploit it. Before he retires, I praise him. He will remain engraved in my heart until my death. He deserves a book-testimony, I agree entirely, and he has my full support. He deserves it.

Conclusion

As a conclusion to this book, I would like to say that I wanted to provide a faithful testimony of this unusual event that occurred in my country with a lot of health, social and economic disruptions. This was an warning to remind us that we must remain prepared to face unexpected humanitarian events.

I wanted to show the efforts made in the fight to reduce the harm done by this disease, to show the value of solidarity, both nationally and internationally, by revealing the power of our unity in the face of a common challenge. When we are united, we can move mountains.

I wanted, through my personal journey, to show the new generation my itinerary full of pitfalls and difficulties, but also to testify to the cardinal values of our society which are, among others, love for the country, commitment to the survival of our society, consolidation of our living together, and perseverance to achieve our goals.

I would like to say that I have remained a peasant and a traditionalist in my perception and love for my national community, knowing that no one can be happy alone and that happiness must be shared with others.

I have great hope that the content of this document will serve humanity, in particular the Guinean nation, in its struggle for human and economic development.

Finally, a griot from Siguiri, in Upper Guinea, sang me the following proverb: "Man can be deprived of his luck". Asking him the meaning of his quotation, he developed in these terms:

1- A successful son who does not care about his parents,

2- A young brother who has everything and leaves his older brother in misery,

3- A rich neighbor who eats to his heart's content and cares little for his neighbors.

This is what it means to be deprived of your chance. To have in one's family, in one's environment, people who can give us a hand and who do not. This is why, as a citizen of Sanankoro, the land where my ancestors were born, I am working to give the best of myself.

Acknowledgements

I cannot end this account of testimonies without expressing my sincere thanks to all those who helped me to put my ideas in order and to help me to express what I wanted to deliver to my readers, in order for them to understand my message and to draw lessons that they will find useful. May these people find here my deep gratitude. I would like to mention in particular some of them, whose contribution was decisive, such as Oumar Sivory Doumbouya, doctor in sociology and teacher-researcher at the University of Toulouse Jean Jaures and at the GLC University of Sonfonia in Conakry, Sansy Kaba, representative of l'Harmattan, Sandrine Segot-Chicq, international technical advisor to myself at ANSS, and Keira Sory, head of the communication department at ANSS. A big thank you to my young brother Aboubacar Nouni Keita, for his contribution to the making of this book.

Annexes

1-LIST OF PEOPLE WHO HAVE DISTINGUISHED THEMSELVES IN THE FIGHT AGAINST EBOLA IN GUINEA

A) Foreign experts

N°	FULL NAME	INSTITUTIONS/NGOs	FUNCTIONS	NATIONALITIES
1	Pr Réné Migliani	French cooperation	Advisor	French
2	Daouda Sissoko	French cooperation	Consultant/Researcher	French
3	Jean Vivient Mombuly	Cooperation Congo Brazzaville	Advisor	Congolese
4	Mohamed Bellhocine	WHO	Representative	Algerian
5	Mamadou Harouna Djingarey	WHO	Deputy Representative	Nigerian
6	Boubacar Diallo	WHO	Epidemiologist	Malian

7	Bruce Aylward Raymond	WHO	WHO Geneva	Canadian
8	Mohamed AG Ayoya	UNICEF	Representative	Malian
9	Seydou Dia	UNICEF	Chief of Emergencies UNICEF	Senegalese
10	GUY Yogo	UNICEF	Deputy Representative	Burkinabé / American
11	Julienne NGOUNDOUNG	UNICEF	Consultant in charge of communication	Cameroonian
12	BOLY Aliou	IFRC	Country Representative	Senegalese
13	Jean Boko KOFFY	IFRC	Chief of Operations	Ivorian
14	OUSMANE FAYE	Pasteur Institute of Dakar	LAB MANAGER	Senegalese
15	Lise Martel	CDC	CDC country director	Canadian/ American
16	Benjamin Dahl	CDC	Epidemiologist	American

17	Pierre Rollin	CDC	Epidemiologist	American/French
18	Tom Frieden	CDC	CDC Director	American
19	Mark Poncin	MSF	MSF Response Coordinator	French
20	Abdou Dieng	UNMEER	Head of UNMEER	Senegalese

B) Guinean experts and national executives

N°	FULL NAME	INSTITUTIONS/ NGOs	FUNCTIONS	Nationalities
1	Mariame Touré	UNICEF		Guinean
2	Mory Condé	UNICEF	NGO AGIL	Guinean
3	Justin Morel Junior	UNICEF	Communication expert	Guinean
4	Abdourahamane Batchily	CNLE	Ebola Coordination Forécariah	Guinean
5	Facinet Yattara	CNLE	Ebola Coordination	Guinean
6	Alexis Traoré	CNLE	Ebola Coordinator Guéckédou	Guinean
7	Aboubacar Moumini Diallo	CNLE	Prefectural Health Director Télémélé and Ebola Coordinator Kérouané	Guinean
8	Facely Diawara	MAF	Head of Health Department CRG	Guinean
9	Youssouf Traoré	MAF	President CRG	Guinean
10	Nouhou DIALLO	MAF	Volunteer	Guinean
11	Mamady KOUROUMA	MAF	Volunteer	Guinean
12	Gnouma Robert KAMANO	MAF	Volunteer	Guinean
13	Barry Moumié	CNLE	Head of Unit Care	Guinean

14	Moussa Konaté	CNLE	Logistics Unit Manager	Guinean
15	Sékou CONDE	CNLE	Assistant National Coordinator	Guinean
16	Sakoba KEITA	CNLE	National Coordinator	Guinean
17	Colonel Rémy Lamah	EX Minister	Health	Guinean
18	Aliouseny Makanéra Kaké	EX Minister	Communication	Guinean
19	Momo CAMARA	CNLE	Area Coordinator	Guinean
20	N'FALLY MAGASSOUBA	LABORATORY hemorrhagic fever	Laboratory Manager	Guinean
21	Lamine Koivogui	National Public Health Institute	Director	Guinean
22	Tata Gackou	Direction Health city Conakry	Director	Guinean
23	Rpland Emanuel Malano	National Directorate for Community Health and Traditional Medicine	Head of Community Health Division	Guinean

CNLE : National Coordination of the Fight against Ebola
GRC : Guinean Red Cross

Postscript: This list is far from exhaustive. Many response workers have also made significant contributions in the field, even to the point of losing their lives. We would like to express our deepest gratitude to them.

2- SPEECH BY THE COORDINATOR OF THE EBOLA RESPONSE UNIT ON THE ASSESSMENT OF THE RESPONSE

Your Excellency the President of the Republic,

Your Excellency the Prime Minister,

Excellencies, Ladies and Gentlemen, Presidents of the Republican Institutions,

Excellencies, members of the government,

Your Excellencies, Ambassadors

Excellencies, representatives of bi and multilateral agencies

Dear guests

Dear companions in the fight against Ebola

It is a great honor for me to stand before you to speak on the Ebola virus disease at the end of this epidemic. Indeed, since the announcement of the results of the tests confirming this disease, on March 21, and the declaration of the epidemic on March 23, 2014, the national health crisis committee, in collaboration with partners, has developed a response plan and set up technical commissions to organize the response. Thus, six commissions were created, namely: surveillance, treatment, communication, logistics, finance, and coordination. This committee was supervised and guided by an inter-ministerial committee. It must be recognized that the knowledge available on the disease at the time did not allow for a better understanding of the complexity of the requirements for an appropriate response. This response had three main strategic stages, namely:

Stage 1, this first phase of the epidemic which extends from January to December 2014 was characterized by the classic response and the mobilization of resources with the help of technical and financial partners. Several elements influenced our efforts to control the epidemic:

- The delay in the mobilization of material and financial resources, logistics, diagnostic means, inputs, and training of agents in management,

- The delay in building Ebola treatment centers,

- Inappropriate messages, rumors, denial, sometimes very violent réticence,

In spite of all these difficulties, thanks to the determination of the various actors in the response, the following results have been achieved in all areas:

1 Treatment: 10 CTEs, 8 CDTs, 3 CTCOMs and 7 laboratories have been set up to provide adequate care.

2 Surveillance: the surveillance system has been strengthened through human resources, computer means and quality data management.

3 Communication: Community mobilization strategies supported by media programs were conducted by community agents, communication experts and socio-anthropologists. Numerous tools have been produced and used and fifteen community radios have been rehabilitated.

4 Logistics: the implementation of logistics was progressive and decisive for the control of the epidemic. Inputs, vehicles, and helicopters were mobilized.

5 Research: Several field studies were conducted on drugs (favipiravir, convalescent plasma, zimap, interferon, etc.), rapid diagnostic test, vaccine trial, follow-up and treatment of survivors. This research has also contributed to the control of the epidemic.

Safe and dignified burials were conducted by Red Cross workers throughout the response, reducing the risk of the disease spreading.

Stage 2, this period from January to June 2015 was characterized by the organization of campaigns: "Ebola Zero in 60 Days," "Ebola is Enough," and action research coupled with awareness raising. These campaigns helped to reduce reluctance and achieve greater community engagement.

Stage 3 covers the period from July to December 2015 and was characterized by the implementation of the cerclage or ring strategy. This was reinforced by the introduction of vaccination, which led to the acceleration of the control of the epidemic. To date the epidemiological situation is as follows:

As of December 29, 2015, we were at:

- Day 43 of the last case's release from the Ebola treatment center,
- Day 46 of the end of contact tracing for the last contact,
- Day 61 of the last positive case notification.

Ladies and gentlemen, it has been a long and arduous process to achieve these results, but thanks to your contributions, we have succeeded. An unprecedented mobilization of financial resources in the fight against the Ebola virus epidemic has been made by the government and its partners. These funds have been used by nearly 53 partners for the purchase of reagents and logistics, construction and rehabilitation of centers, staff motivation and various operating expenses.

This journey has instructed and inspired us to develop roadmaps and operational action plans to provide corrective solutions to identified weaknesses. These plans, which are part of the Ministry of Health's re-launch, provide hope for strengthening the health system by making it capable of quickly controlling any epidemic as soon as it appears.

No.	Categories	Cases	Deaths
1	Confirmed cases	3351	2083
2	Probable cases	453	453
3	Suspected cases	0	0
4	Total	3804	2536
5	Healthcare workers	211	115
6	Healed / discharged	1268	

It is within this framework that we invite all actors to set up a functional rapid response mechanism in early 2016.

Ladies and Gentlemen, I would like to express my deepest gratitude to the partners, the members of the government, the members of the national, regional, and district coordination teams for their contribution in the conduct and management of this response.

Your Excellency, Mr. President, I cannot find the words to express to you the deep feelings I have after completing this task. All the honors that I have received during this response are due to you, you have allowed me to express myself and to make myself known on the national and international level. I thank you for this and send you my deepest gratitude.

My response team remains at your disposal to accompany you on the path of building our country for its development.

TOGETHER WE DEFEATED EBOLA, GOODBYE EBOLA.

Thank you.

3- SPEECH BY PROFESSOR RENÉ MIGLIANI, CNRE ADVISOR

Public health professor sent by the French government to support the management and coordination of the Ebola response in Guinea.

Mr. President,

I thank you for this dinner in my honor. I am sincerely touched by your attention. Personally, I am leaving Guinea after nine months of presence, of struggles rich in meetings, exchanges, and rare moments in a professional and human life.

How can I forget this shared adventure? It is impossible and my memory will never fail me, even if Alzheimer's catches up with me. I don't have enough time to say a word to all of you but know that you are in my heart.

If I had to choose one, without hesitation, my choice would be the national coordinator, Dr. Sakoba Keïta, with whom we have built a friendship over time, events and our many missions in the field.

Yes, the national coordination has often gone to the field. Through our exchanges, our common meals made of rice, fish and spicy sauces that the Soussous are so fond of, the little sandwiches prepared by Mrs. Sakoba during our missions. We have more than built, we have knitted a true friendship with the only objective, the fight against the Ebola virus. I can and want to say that Guinea has been lucky to have in Sakoba a rare treasure, full of experience, intelligence, common sense, charisma, rigor, and uncommon resistance.

As I said to him sometimes: "If Guinea had had twenty-five Sakoba, many things would have changed". For all these reasons, I personally award him the title of "Professor Keïta".

Mr. President, allow me to conclude my speech on these words and I thank you again for the opportunity you have given me to accompany you in the fight against the Ebola epidemic, while wishing your beautiful country to end this epidemic very quickly.

June 27, 2015

Professor René MIGLIANI.

4- CREATION OF THE EBOLA MUSEUM AT THE NATIONAL AGENCY FOR HEALTH SECURITY (ANSS)

RULES OF PROCEDURE FOR VISITORS TO THE EBOLA NATIONAL MUSEUM

As part of the fixation for the collective memory, the National Agency for Health Security (ANSS), heir of the National Coordination Unit for the fight against Ebola (CNLE), through the Department of Communication and Social Mobilization, has opened an exhibition-preservation space of works retracing the dark period of the epidemic of this pathology in the Republic of Guinea: **The Ebola Museum**.

In order to allow posterity to live, if only in memory of the brave struggle led by Guinea and its partners, ANSS has established a certain number of rules or principles to be respected by any visitor to the site.

The **Ebola Museum** is located on the 3rd floor of the "Pita" building.

The present document, known as the Rules of Procedure, is hereby adopted and is structured as follows:

Title 1: Preamble
Title 2: Scope of Application
Title 3: Access to the Museum
Title 4: Locker room - objects
Title 5: General conduct of visitors
Title 6: Photography, recording, copying and reprography
Title 7: Use of the Internet in the Museum
Title 8: Safety of persons, works and buildings
Title 9: Enforcement

PREAMBLE

Area of competence of the museum's internal regulations

These rules and regulations apply to :

0. ANSS managers and officers
1. External persons

In the interest of sustainable management of the museum, visitors are expected to comply with the provisions of these rules.

The museum's spaces are open to the public and include:

- Reception area
- Space for the presentation of the permanent collections.

REGULATORY PROVISIONS APPLICABLE TO VISITORS

It is strictly forbidden for visitors to:

- **Touch or take, with the intention of taking with oneself, therefore, stealing, any object of the museum;**
- Destroy or intentionally damage any listed or registered object and any piece of furniture in the museum's pavilions;
- Unauthorized entry into the museum outside of set hours;
- Eat or bring food into the museum;
- Smoking in the museum;
- Wear an outfit that may conceal your face

ACCESS TO THE MUSEUM

The regular opening days and hours of the museum are Monday, from 8:00 am to 4:30 pm to Friday, from 8:00 am to 4:30 pm, except for public holidays.

The closing of the museum to the public can be decided according to exceptional measures of the General Direction of the ANSS.

Any attempt to close the museum will be the subject of a memo from the DG or his deputy in which the reason for and time frame of the closure will be defined.

The visit of the museum is conditioned to the possession of an access badge. No access will be allowed in the museum without a badge.

The access badge is issued to the visitor who requests it from the museum administrator. It will be recorded in a register dedicated to this purpose.

LOCKER-OBJECT

Objects whose presence does not seem compatible with the security of the museum may be rejected by the administrator.

The Agency declines all responsibility in the event of loss of an object by a visitor that has not been reported at the museum entrance. However, **a locker is available free of charge to users.**

Any object of a suspicious nature found on a visitor inside the museum will be handed over to the competent authority for possible decision.

GENERAL VISITOR BEHAVIOR

It is strictly forbidden for any visitor to enter the museum with:

1. Weapons, ammunition, explosive substances, in short, any dangerous object;
2. Animals with the exception of the motor or visual handicapped and whose company requires these animals;
3. Bulky items (suitcase, large bag, briefcase and luggage) ;
4. Commercial photography ;
5. Camera for filming the premises if not authorized.
6. Journalists may be authorized, in exceptional circumstances, by the museum administrator, to film and take pictures with flashes or artificial light during or outside public opening hours.
7. Visitors are expected to comply with any remarks made by the museum administrator for service or ethical reasons.

Failure to comply with these rules and regulations may result in the visitor being excluded from the museum and, where appropriate, being liable to pay compensation for any damage caused to an object in the museum.

USE OF THE INTERNET

It is strictly forbidden inside the museum to use:

- Pornographic site
- Sites that promote violence, discrimination, or any other illegal practice.

SECURITY OF PEOPLE AND THE MUSEUM

The visiting public is informed that for security reasons, the museum premises are under video surveillance (camera).

For everyone's safety, visitors must comply with the security measures proposed by the museum administrator.

Any visitor who witnesses a case of theft is asked to alert the museum administrator for disciplinary action.

The museum administrator is responsible for the strict enforcement of these rules and regulations.

These rules and regulations are posted on a board at the front of the museum for your information.

Conakry, March ____ 2017
The head of the Communication Department
and Social Mobilization

Approved by the Deputy Director General of the ANSS

Approved by the DG of the ANSS

5- THE 9 DECLARATIONS DURING EBOLA IN GUINEA

Viral hemorrhagic fever epidemic in Guinea: Statement by the Minister of Health,

Conakry, March 21, 2014

Since February 9, 2014, our country has recorded cases of febrile illnesses in some prefectures of Forest Guinea and Conakry. To date, 49 cases of febrile illnesses, including 29 deaths, have been recorded.

These cases were recorded in the prefectures of Guéckédou, Macenta, Kissidougou and in Conakry. This disease manifests itself by an outbreak of fever, diarrhea, vomiting, pronounced fatigue and sometimes bleeding.

Faced with this situation, the Ministry of Health, in collaboration with its partners, sent a rapid investigation mission to the field to determine the nature of this disease. The first results confirm the presence of a virus responsible for hemorrhagic fevers.

This disease, which has already caused a significant number of deaths, is transmitted mainly from sick to healthy people and through soiled objects belonging to sick or dead people. Also, the consumption of meat from infected bush animals can be a source of contamination.

THIS SITUATION LEADS THE GOVERNMENT TO MAKE THE PRESENT DECLARATION OF AN EPIDEMIC OF

HEMORRHAGIC VIRAL FEVER IN GUINEA.

As a result, the Department of Health has taken the following actions:

- Free treatment for all patients in isolation centers,
- Informing the population about individual and collective hygiene measures,
- Exclusive responsibility for the treatment of the bodies of deceased patients to health personnel and the Guinean Red Cross, to limit contamination,
- Identification of all persons who have had direct contact with the deceased and those with the signs mentioned above,
- Dissemination of awareness messages in the media (radio, TV, internet).

Ladies and gentlemen, the government, in this period of epidemic, invites:

Health Services:

a. to take all necessary steps to inform the medical staff about the preventive measures and treatment of this disease;

b. to report any suspected cases to the Disease Prevention and Control Division;

c. to inform the patients and their families about individual and collective hygiene measures;

To the people:

a. to keep their serenity, because adequate measures are taken for the control of this disease;

b. report any suspected cases to the nearest health authority;

c. the practice of individual and collective hygiene measures, which are sanitation of the premises, hand washing with soap and chlorine or bleach.

The government expresses its satisfaction to the partners for their support since the beginning of this epidemic and takes the opportunity to count on the actions they will carry out at our side for the control and eradication of this disease.

Thank you.

Colonel Remy Lamah, MD

Ebola Fever Epidemic
Statement No. 2 from the Minister of Health, Doctor-Colonel Rémy Lama

As you know, our country, Guinea, is experiencing an Ebola outbreak declared on March 21, 2014.

Since then, many actions have been undertaken by the government, with the support of partners, to curb this disease, which occurred for the first time in Guinea.

In my first statement, dated March 21, 2014, I had, among other measures, asked the population to practice individual and collective hygiene measures including hand washing.

I am sorry to see and to receive information about the abusive and even dangerous use of chlorine solution and bleach.

I would like to inform you all that it has recently been proven that the Ebola virus does not resist proper hand washing with soap and water, without the addition of chlorine or bleach. Fortunately, the Ebola virus is very fragile. I urge you to practice careful and regular hand washing with soap and water to prevent hand-to-mouth transmission.

Let's reserve the use of chlorine or bleach in the right dosage, I insist on the right dosage, depending on the degree of people who have died of Ebola, are suspected, or have had contact with confirmed patients. This mission of disinfection of homes is entrusted to the Guinean Red Cross.

Chlorine solution or bleach should also be used for cleaning vegetables and fruits.

We must also use it for the treatment of drinking water, again with a good dosage. One capful of chlorine solution for 20 liters of water, or two capfuls when the water is cloudy. This practice should be repeated every day because water treated the day before is not drinkable after 24 hours.

For cooking foods, proper cooking is enough to destroy the Ebola virus.

Improperly used chlorine solution or bleach can be dangerous to health and have irreversible consequences that can even lead to death.

Avoid misuse. Seek advice from pharmacists, health workers, Red Cross volunteers, and anyone else you trust who can read and tell you the correct dosage of chlorine solution or bleach.

Dear compatriots, I reiterate my call for serenity because the actions taken to control this disease are producing reassuring results.

The government thanks the partners for their constant support since the beginning of this epidemic in Guinea.

Together, we will defeat this epidemic.

Thank you.

MESSAGE TO THE NATION FROM THE PRESIDENT OF THE REPUBLIC, HEAD OF STATE, Prof. ALPHA CONDÉ, ON THE EBOLA HEMORRHAGIC FEVER EPIDEMIC

Conakry, March 30, 2014

Guineans and Guineans. Dear compatriots!

First and foremost, I would like to ask everyone to observe a minute of silence in memory of our compatriots who have died as a result of Ebola.

Dear compatriots,

As you know, Guinea, our country, is currently facing an Ebola viral hemorrhagic fever epidemic. To date, 116 patients have been registered, of whom 72 have died, including health workers. The government sends its sincere condolences to the bereaved families.

As soon as this epidemic was announced, **I instructed the government, which took important measures to fight this disease, which is a health emergency. It is within this framework that I particularly instructed the Minister of Health who issued a statement on March 21, 2014 to inform the population and the international community.**

Dear compatriots,

In my capacity as President of the Republic, Head of State, **my government and I are very concerned about the epidemic, which affects the most active sectors of the country, including health workers.**

This is why **I would like to reassure the population that, thanks to the support of the international community, all measures are being taken to effectively fight this epidemic.**

I **strongly appeal to the population to strictly respect the preventive measures given by the health services through the different messages.**

I also ask the population not to give in to panic, nor to believe rumors.

Dear compatriots and foreigners who live among us, I invite you to be more serene. Because, in addition to the Guinean health personnel that I would like to congratulate and encourage, Guinea is currently benefiting from an unprecedented mobilization of several specialists to help us defeat this disease.

I have instructed prefects, governors, mayors, and CRD presidents to work very closely with international partners on the ground so that Guinea can defeat this epidemic very quickly.

I ask the elders and the populations, at all levels, to facilitate the task of the health personnel and the specialists who have come to help our country.

Finally, I would like to sincerely thank the international community for its mobilization and support in the fight against Ebola hemorrhagic fever in Guinea.

May God bless Guinea and Guineans. Amen!

Thank you.

President Alpha Condé declares a national health emergency

Statement : "Our country is facing an Ebola virus disease epidemic, since the beginning of this year. Faced with this situation, the international community has mobilized strongly by organizing many strategic meetings, including the summit of heads of state of the Mano River Union, the summit of heads of state of Africa and the United States in Washington, and the meeting in Geneva.

At the end of these meetings, it became clear that the disease situation is critical and threatens the health of many countries in the world.

For these reasons, the WHO has declared a global health emergency against the Ebola virus disease.

- Considering that Guinea is a signatory member of the World Health Organization constitution;
- In view of Law 97/021/AN of June 19, 1997, on the Public Health Code, which has as its fundamental principle to ensure the protection and promotion of the health of individuals, families and communities in the Republic of Guinea;
- In view of the provisions relating to the management of epidemics,

I hereby declare a national health emergency for the Ebola virus disease in the Republic of Guinea.

In this context, and in addition to those already stated in my statement of March 30, the following measures are prescribed

1) A **health cordon** manned by health, security and defense officials is established at all border crossings into the Republic of Guinea.

2) The movement of people is restricted and subject to **health control measures** at the various land, sea and airport crossing points.

3) All health, security and defense personnel are mobilized to fight the disease.

4) All ministerial departments, private sector actors and civil society are invited to join the fight against the disease in the areas of awareness and prevention.

5) All suspected cases will be **routinely sampled** and hospitalized until laboratory results are available.

6) All contacts are strictly forbidden to move outside their area of residence until the end of their surveillance period.

7) The **transfer of bodies** from one locality to another is **prohibited** until the end of the epidemic.

8) **The systematic use of protective equipment** is instituted **in all public and private health structures** in the country.

9) **Any person who opposes or incites opposition in any way to the detection, treatment, isolation or examination of a patient, suspect or contact shall be considered a threat to the public health and shall be subject to the full force of the law.**

The response committees at the national, prefectural, and sub-prefectural levels are instructed to conduct a daily assessment of the situation and share information with national and international actors and partners.

These measures are effective as of this 13th day of August 2014."

Conakry, August 13, 2014

Pr Alpha CONDÉ
President of the Republic
Head of State

FORUM OF THE FORCES VIVES OF GUINEA AGAINST EBOLA

Conakry, March 12, 2015

== STATEMENT ==

While Ebola continues to strike hard at our mothers, fathers, brothers and sisters, dramatically mourning our dear country, our Guinea, threatening its destiny,

We, the youth of a united and fraternal Guinea,

Thank you, all of you, here present, representatives of Guinean society, in all its components; political parties, religious and traditional leaders, civil society in all its diversity; for having made the commitment to join forces to preserve our country and our future, for a happy and prosperous Guinea free of the Ebola virus disease.

On this memorable day, we say that this commitment is based on principles, namely:

- First - The Ebola epidemic is recognized as a national challenge and a priority until all cases in Guinea and neighboring countries are eliminated;

- Second - The Guinean nation, in all its components, commits to a national consensus for the Ebola response;

- Third - This national unity against Ebola is above all the socio-political cleavages existing in the country, especially in this post-colonial period;

- Fourthly - All of Guinea's stakeholders are participating in and supporting, in the same spirit of solidarity, the remarkable action of national and international actors in the prevention and fight against the spread of the epidemic;

and

- Fifth - In this dynamic of national mobilization, rumors and false information that destabilize the work of the response teams and affect the effectiveness of their intervention must be banished.

Together, on the basis of these fundamental principles, let us ensure that Guinea sets an example in its fight against Ebola, and let us stand together until the last patient is healed.

Declaration of a reinforced health emergency by the President of the Republic, Pr Alpha Condé

Saturday, March 28, 2015

Guinean women,
Guineans,
Dear compatriots,

I come before you today to discuss the progress of the Ebola epidemic facing our country.

As you know, on August 13, 2014, I had signed the declaration of a national health emergency in our country. At the time, the epidemic was out of control and was claiming more and more victims throughout the country.

Since then, 3,478 Guineans have been affected and 1,880 have died. Health personnel have paid a heavy price, with 200 health workers infected and 108 dead.

The general evolution of the crisis management allows us to note notable improvements:

The prefectures of Forest Guinea have been Ebola-free for 21 days: 0 cases of illness, 0 contacts.

The technical means, mobile laboratories and others allow to reduce the time to obtain the test results.

The population is becoming increasingly aware, and the last pockets of reluctance are disappearing.

A new school year has begun without incident. Students are better informed and more engaged in the fight against Ebola.

Today, 54 confirmed cases and 26 suspected cases are being treated at the various treatment centers.

The number of people recovering from Ebola is increasing and their return to their families is an encouraging sign.

Guineans, Guineans,

What has been done is important. What remains to be done is critical and vital.

As the epidemic experts say, it is easier to go from 100 to 10 than from 10 to 0. That is, what we have left to do is more difficult than what we have already done.

However, I regret to note that there is a growing abandonment of vigilance and precautions that are essential to save the lives of our populations. All the measures decreed by the declaration of health emergency and the recommendations of the national coordination of the fight against Ebola are less and less followed.

This culpable negligence is manifesting itself at the very heart of our health care system. A department in a local hospital and several private clinics have been affected by the virus. It is extremely difficult that health personnel, who have paid a high price for this epidemic, are vectors instead of bulwarks.

The mapping of the epidemic, today, has moved to the coast of our country, in the prefectures of Forécariah, Coyah, Kindia, Dubréka and Boffa. In this densely populated area, the epidemic represents a real risk for the health of our nation.

That is why I am declaring a reinforced health emergency for the prefectures of Forécariah, Coyah, Dubréka, Boffa and Kindia for a period of 45 days. In Conakry, rigorous measures will also be taken in the localities.

The following measures must be taken and strictly enforced:

- Hospitals and private clinics where cases of Ebola have been reported should be temporarily closed; patients already in the hospital or clinic should remain there and arrangements will be made for their care and feeding.

- Other health care facilities that do not implement the prevention measures should also be closed.

- All cases of death during this period of heightened health emergency must be systematically tested.

- All burials in the area covered by the enhanced health emergency must be secured in advance by the Red Cross or Civil Defence, with respect for human dignity.

- Burial, mourning, and condolence ceremonies should be kept to a minimum; greetings and ritual gatherings may be postponed beyond the period of heightened health emergency.

- Any person who hides patients or moves bodies from one locality to another will be prosecuted, according to the law, for endangering the lives of others.

- Accompaniment and support measures for families and health workers must be reinforced by the national coordination of the fight against Ebola.

- The Minister of Health must intensify supervision of health care facilities and ensure compliance with preventive measures.

Wherever necessary, during this health emergency, containment and confinement measures will be taken and efforts will be made to provide food and health support to the affected populations.

All ministerial departments, regions, prefectures, and communes, as well as health establishments and structures, must ensure the strict application of these measures.

Guineans, Guineans,

The Ebola epidemic is imposing an extremely difficult test on our country and our brothers and sisters in Sierra Leone and Liberia.

I call on society's organizations, political parties, local elected officials, trade unions, the media, youth, and women to mobilize and commit themselves to the fight against Ebola.

Ebola is not over, but it can be over quickly if we follow these steps.

For the future of our nation, we must, here and now, demonstrate courage, sacrifice, and discipline.

May God bless Guinea. Amen!

Pr. Alpha Condé
President of the Republic
Head of State

Heads of State of Guinea and Sierra Leone to meet in Pamelap on June 5
Declaration of a heightened and extended health emergency

The Heads of State of Guinea and Sierra Leone, concerned about the health of their populations and determined to put an end to the Ebola virus disease epidemic, met on June 5, 2015 in Gbalamouya (Pamelap, Forécariah prefecture) to harmonize their points of view in the implementation of a strategy to strengthen and extend the measures contained in the memorandum of understanding signed between the administrative authorities and the response actors of the two border towns of Forécariah and Kambia on March 26, 2015.

Following the persistence of the Ebola epidemic in some areas of Guinea and Sierra Leone, despite numerous meetings between the Heads of State of the Mano River and technical teams extended to partners, it was noted that the bottleneck of the response remains the low commitment of the populations and authorities in some localities of the two countries.

At the end of the meeting, the two Heads of State, Prof. Aplha Condé and Enest Baï Koroma, agreed to extend the reinforced health emergency measures in their respective countries until June 30, 2015.

These measures are:

1 - Hospitals and private clinics where Ebola cases have been reported should be temporarily closed. Patients already in these facilities must remain in place and measures will be taken to ensure their treatment and feeding;

2 - Other health care facilities that do not apply preventive measures must also be closed;

3 - Any healer or traditional therapist who does not refer Ebola suspects to specialized health structures will be prosecuted for endangering the lives of others;

4 - Any religious leader who does not observe the measures enacted or who incites denial of the Ebola disease will be prosecuted by the law in force;

5 - All cases of death during this period of heightened health emergency must be systematically tested;

6 - All burials in the area covered by the enhanced health emergency must be secured in advance by the Red Cross or civil protection, with respect for human dignity;

7 - Burial, mourning and condolence ceremonies should be kept to the strictest privacy of the family setting. Ritual greetings and gatherings may be postponed beyond the period of heightened health emergency.

8 - Any person who hides sick people or moves bodies from one locality to another shall be considered a criminal who spreads disease and shall be prosecuted, in accordance with the law, for endangering the lives of others.

9 - Any person who threatens or attacks the actors of the response, their equipment or public and private buildings will be prosecuted and severely punished by law;

10 - Response teams are encouraged to propose new initiatives to search for and eliminate all residual Ebola cases in all remaining active locations;

11 - Technical and financial partners are invited to support the effective implementation of these measures;

12 - The local administrative authorities have full powers for the strict and rigorous application of these measures;

13 - The defense and security forces are invited to take all necessary measures for the strict application of the present measures;

14 - Exceptional movement restriction measures will be applied to locations with contacts;

15 - Accompaniment and support measures for families and health workers must be reinforced by the national coordination of the fight against Ebola;

16 - The Minister of Health shall intensify the supervision of health care facilities and ensure compliance with preventive measures.

The Guinean prefectures affected by this declaration of a heightened health emergency are: **Forécariah, Coyah, Dubréka, Boké, Kindia, Boffa, Fria and the city of Conakry.**

All the ministerial departments concerned (Health, Territorial Administration, Education, Security, Justice, Religious Affairs, Communication...) are invited, each in its own area, to respect the effective application of this declaration.

Done in Gbalamouya (Forécariah) on June 5, 2015

DECLARATION CEREMONY OF THE END OF THE TRANSMISSION OF THE EBOLA VIRUS EPIDEMIC IN GUINEA

Statement by Prof. Mohammed Belhocine
WHO Representative,

Conakry, December 29, 2015

Ladies and Gentlemen

As we speak, this December 29, 2015, forty-two days have passed since the newborn and last confirmed Ebola case was released from the disease treatment unit in Nongo, Conakry.

This little girl's heroic body overcame the disease, helped by the treatment administered by a very dedicated and professional team.

The criteria established by the World Health Organization to declare the end of all known Ebola transmission in Guinea has been met.

The Ebola outbreak in Guinea is over.

— **Ndénaonaré Ébola la Guinè, lanni (Poular)**

— **Djankaro mèntö Ébola baraban**, la Guinè (Maninka)

— **Fouré nakhar khili Ébola baranion, la Guinè (Sosso)**

— **Ebola a ak'pé laminé, (Kpèlè)**

It is an understatement to say that this epidemic has caused serious disruptions in the economic and social life of the country. Almost all sectors of activity have been affected.

The health sector has suffered serious consequences in terms of the use of essential services. It has paid a heavy price through the professionals who have died trying to save the lives of their fellow human beings. Education, air transport, mining activities, economic exchanges, pilgrimage to Mecca have all been negatively affected by this situation.

At the height of the epidemic in November 2014, the country was recording hundreds of cases per week. The social fabric was strained. Communities, families, and individuals were marked by disbelief, fear, uncertainty of tomorrow, the shock of multiple bereavements in a very short time.

In this context, having succeeded in interrupting the transmission of this deadly virus is a huge national success.

The government and the people of Guinea are to be commended.

In the face of adversity, they have managed to stand up and fight the epidemic with courage and selflessness. We must also salute the pioneering and visionary character of the acceptance of clinical trials for a new vaccine and certain treatments.

Health, social and community mobilization professionals, volunteers, civil society organizations, communities and security services all demonstrated a high sense of solidarity, responsibility, and commitment. The international community has not been left out in its moral, material, technical and financial support.

The experience gained should not be lost now that the respite of the end of the epidemic is here.

We know that the virus is formidable and capable of resurgence. Recent history in a neighboring country has reminded us of this.

Another 90 days of reinforced epidemiological surveillance, the maintenance of a solid investigation capacity, the implementation of a rapid response plan, the care of those recovered from Ebola, and the revival of the health system are the best guarantees to prevent new epidemic outbreaks. The government is working on this, and the international community is committed to supporting it.

The World Health Organization, with its partners, will continue to fulfill its mandate and support all these efforts.

On behalf of the WHO Director General, Dr. Margaret Chan, and the Regional Director for Africa, Dr. Matshidio Moeti, I would like to express our sincere congratulations to the people and government of Guinea for this phenomenal success.

Thank you.

WHO declares end of 2nd Ebola outbreak

"On this day, June 1, 2016, I declare, on behalf of the World Health Organization (WHO), the end of the Ebola virus disease that occurred on March 17, 2016 in the prefecture of N'Nzérékoré and Macenta. The last case released from the Ebola treatment center in Nzérékoré was declared cured 42 days ago, the time frame recommended by WHO to declare the end of the Ebola virus disease epidemic.

However, everyone should keep in mind **that as of today, the 90-day period of enhanced surveillance recommended by the WHO begins to ensure that any outbreak is immediately detected before transmission to others**. Vigilance, as well as response capabilities, will need to be maintained.

WHO encourages the Minister of Health, the National Ebola Coordination, and technical and financial partners to support ongoing priority interventions, including:

– Active surveillance in a belt (the SA Ceint) centered around those recovered from Ebola with their own participation. There is now evidence that the disease virus can survive in some organs of people who have recovered from Ebola for more than 15 months. So, we need to strengthen surveillance and vaccination around recovered people, with their own participation.

– The implementation of integrated disease surveillance and response (IDSR) This surveillance aims to detect, notify and confirm any epidemic or health emergency at an early stage so that it can be rapidly controlled, thus avoiding any risk of the disease spreading.

In addition to these various measures, a rapid response mechanism has been set up in Guinea, under the aegis of the WHO, in collaboration with the health authorities and all partners, to ensure an effective and coordinated response to any health emergency in the country.

We also need to remind people to maintain the good practices they have learned in terms of individual and collective hygiene.

WHO is working with the governments of Guinea, Liberia, and Sierra Leone, the three most affected countries, to strengthen their health systems and priority health programs, while continuing to maintain capacity to detect, prevent, and respond to any Ebola outbreak.

On behalf of the WHO Director General, **Dr Margaret Chan**, and the Regional Director for Africa, **Dr Matshidiso Moeti,** I would like to express our sincere congratulations to the people and government of Guinea, and all partners, for their unity of action in containing this outbreak. »

Dr. Abou Beckr GAYE, acting WHO representative in Guinea.

Photos

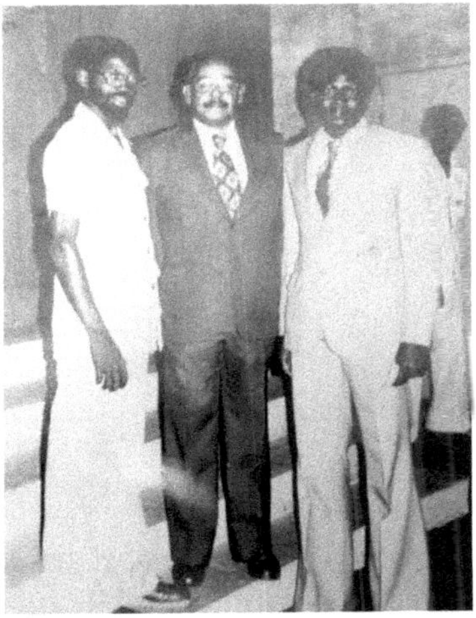

Graduation in 19809 with Professor Juan Pabtiste Ortega and Abdoulaye Katia Camara

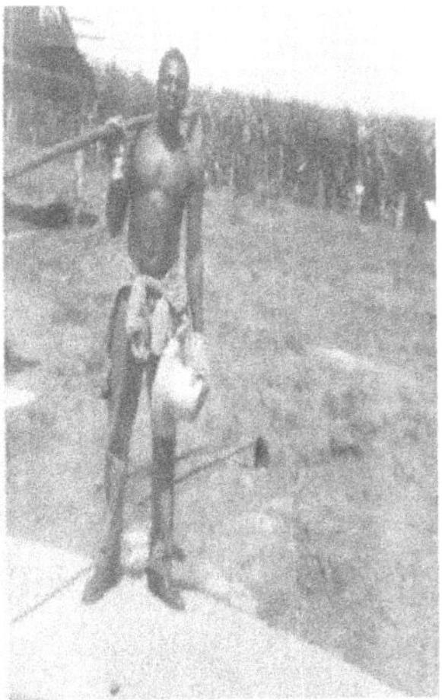

Voluntary field work in 1975

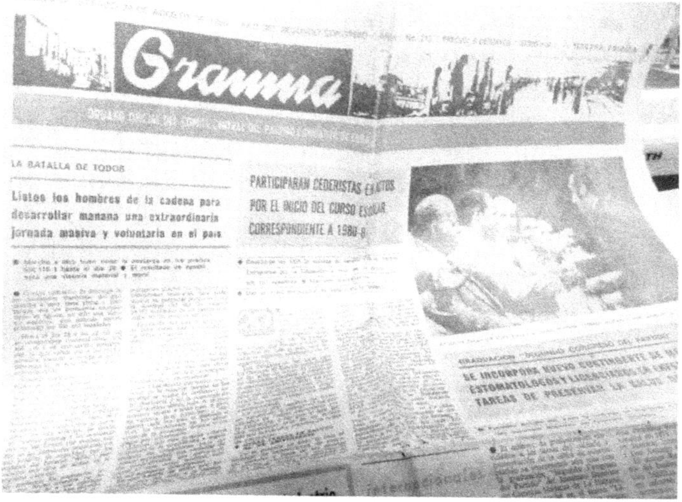

Granma

LA BATALLA DE TODOS

Listos los hombres de la cadena para desarrollar mañana una extraordinaria jornada masiva y voluntaria en el país

PARTICIPARAN CEDERISTAS EN ACTOS POR EL INICIO DEL CURSO ESCOLAR CORRESPONDIENTE A 1980-8

Graduation journal which designates the author as the best foreign student of his class

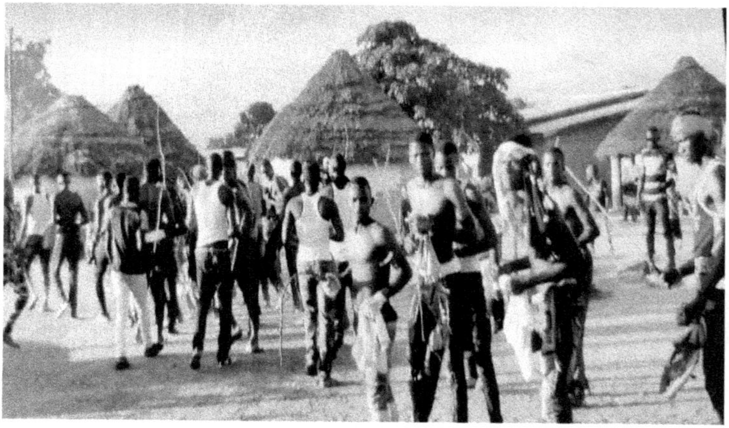

Meeting with the elders of the village of Sanankoro (Kouroussa)

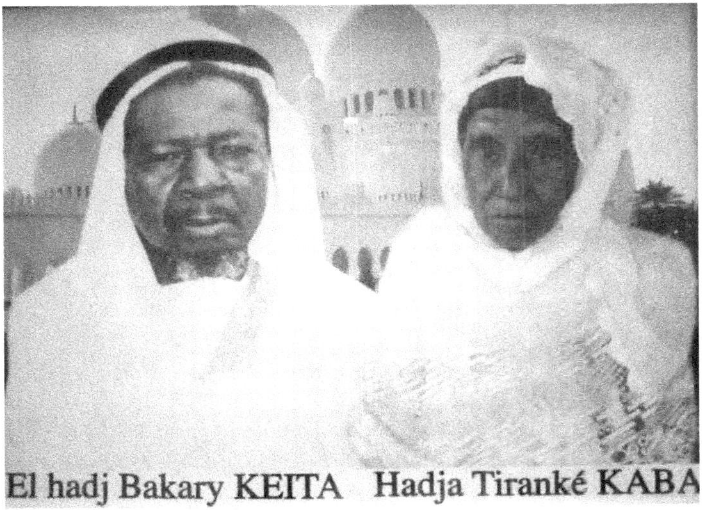

The parents of the author

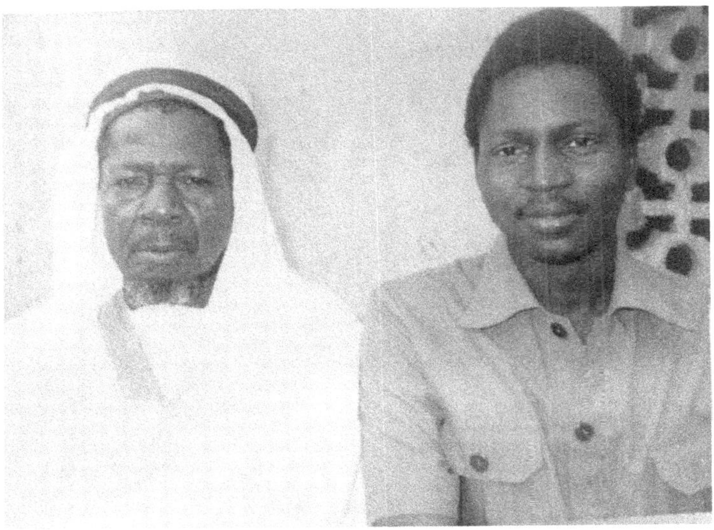

The author and his father in 1982

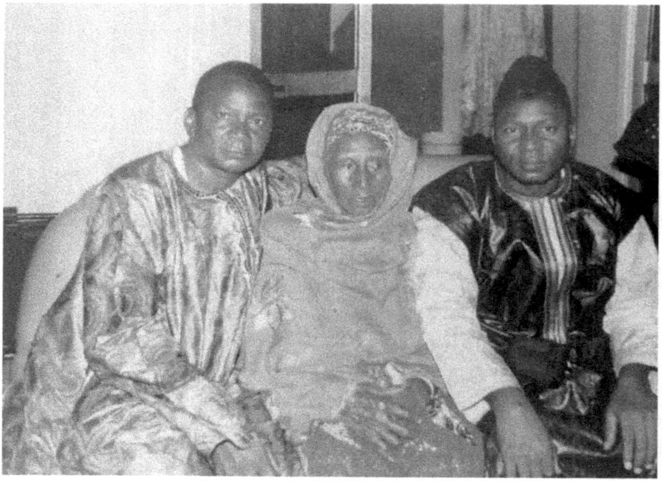

Picture of the author with his mother (Tiranke Kaba) and his young brother Mamadi Keita

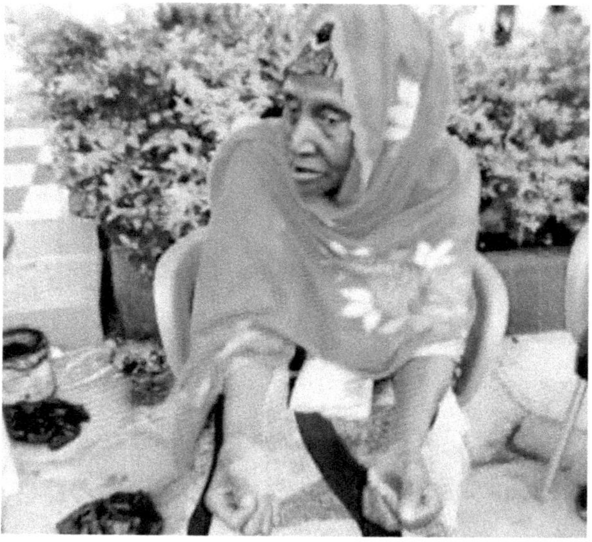

The author's mother's blessings

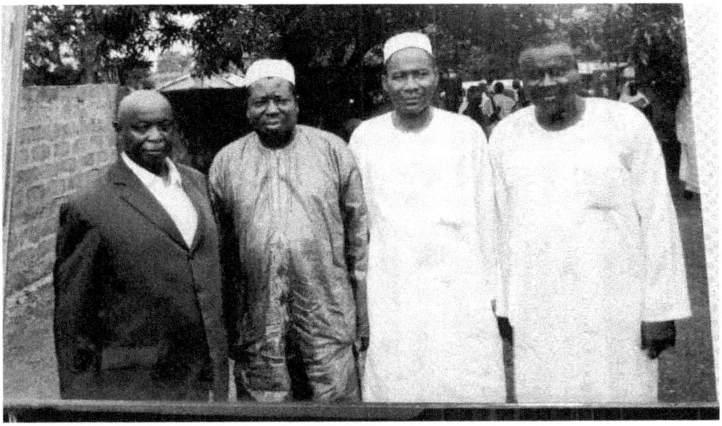

The author's cousins

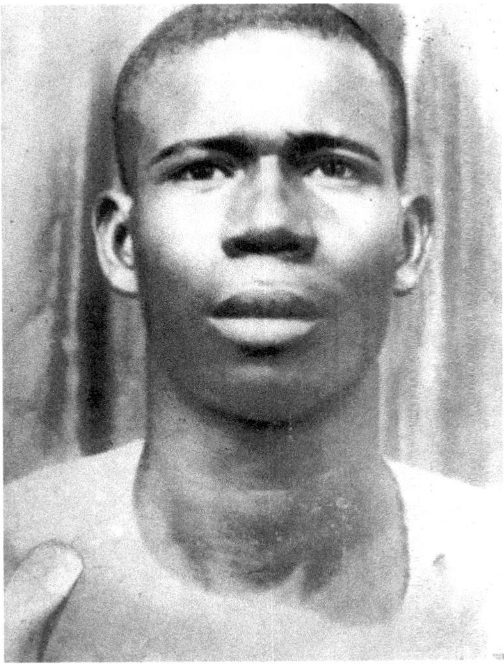

Uncle of the author, his tutor in Conakry

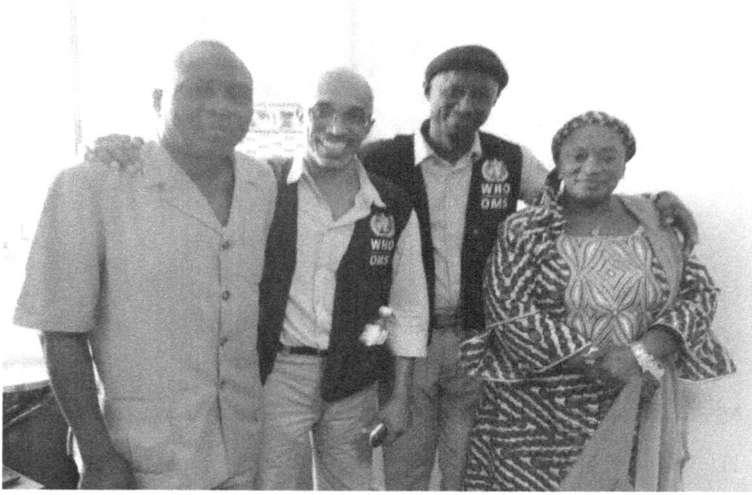

In company of a WHO team

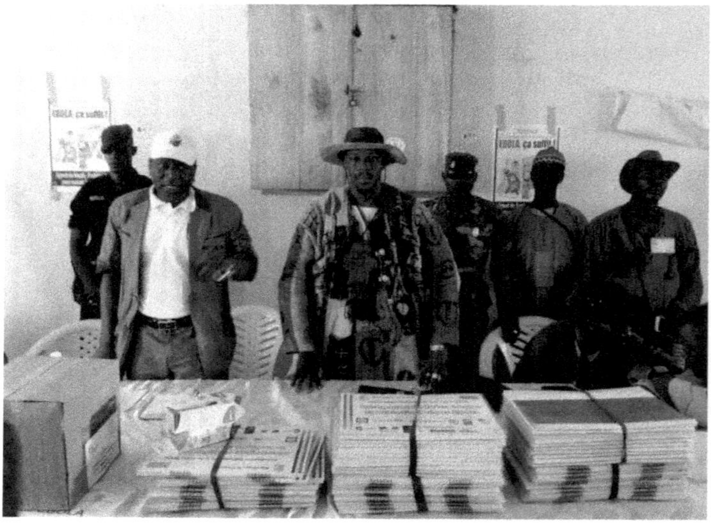

In company of traditional healers

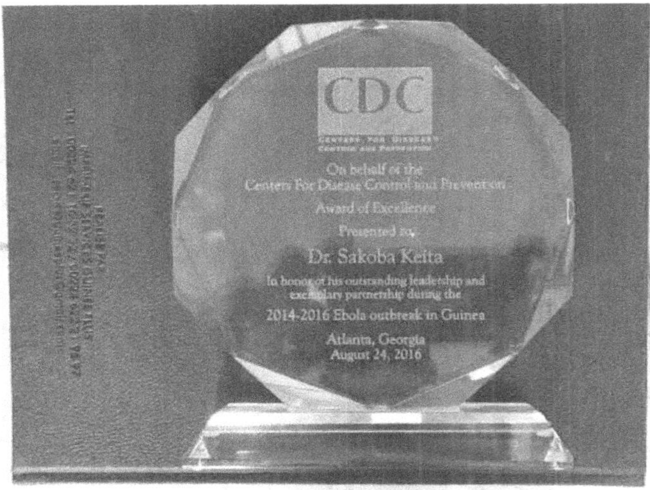
CDC
On behalf of the
Centers For Disease Control and Prevention
Award of Excellence
Presented to
Dr. Sakoba Keita
2014-2016 Ebola outbreak in Guinea
Atlanta, Georgia
August 24, 2016

CDC recognition for best epidemiologist in 2016
in Atlanta

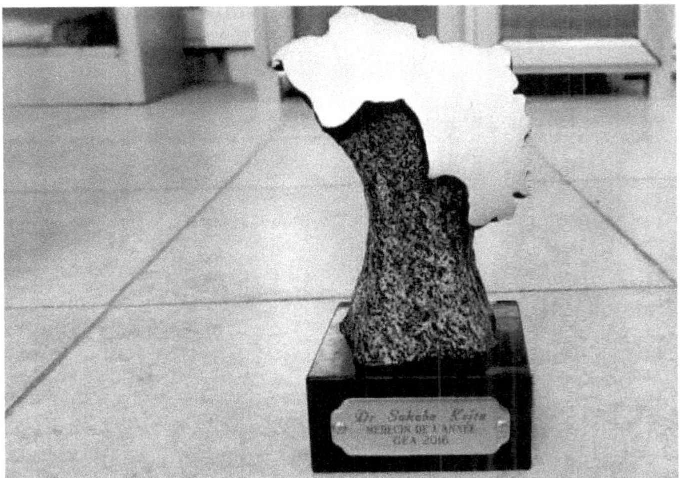
Dr Sakoba Keita

Distinction from Guineans in Canada

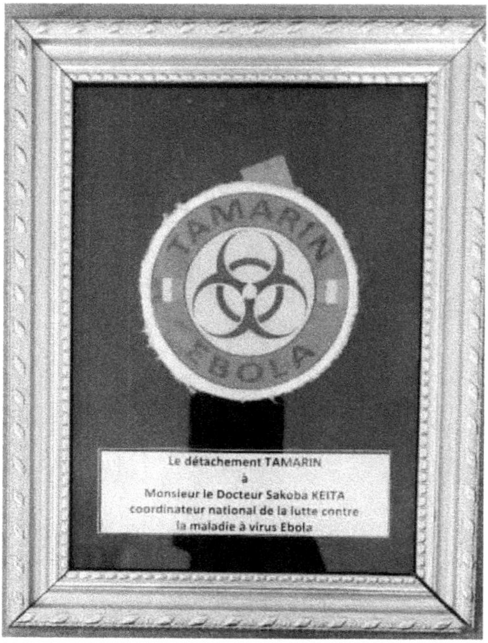
TAMARIN
EBOLA
Le détachement TAMARIN
à
Monsieur le Docteur Sakoba KEITA
coordinateur national de la lutte contre
la maladie à virus Ebola

Other distinction

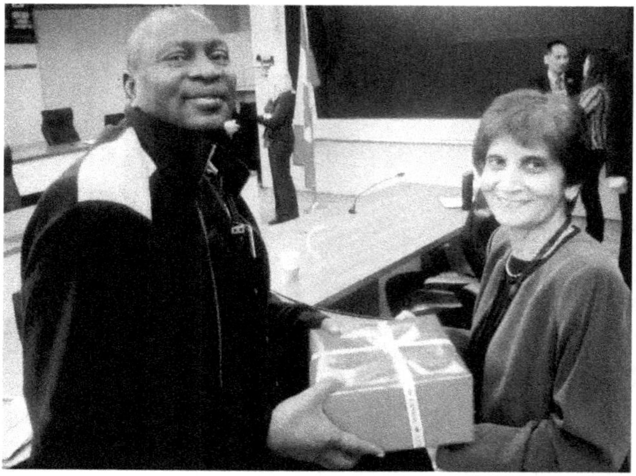

Recognition by Public Health Canada

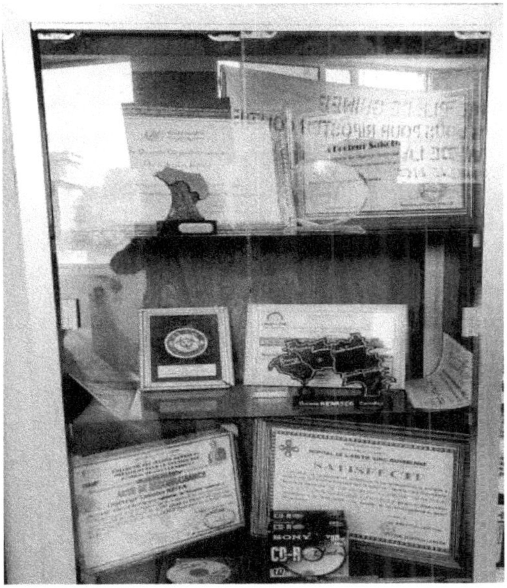

Certificates of satisfaction from different NGOs

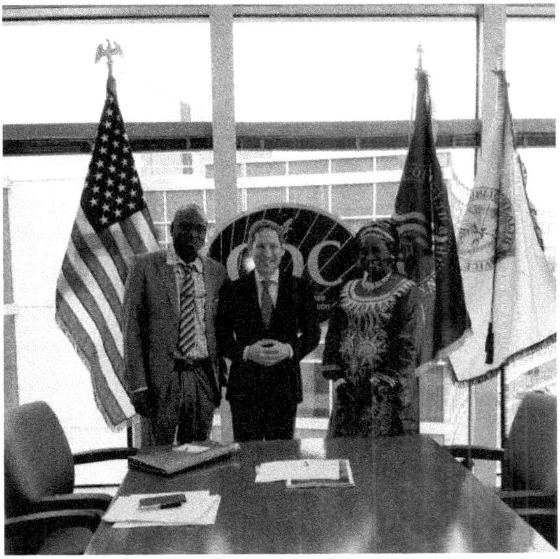

With Tom Frieden, ex-director of CDC-Atlanta

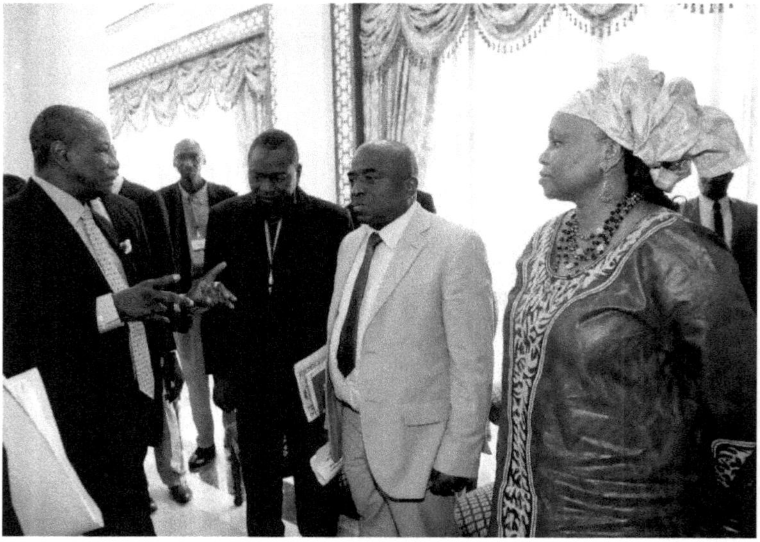

During During a donation ceremony with ministers Remy Lamah and Rougui Barry

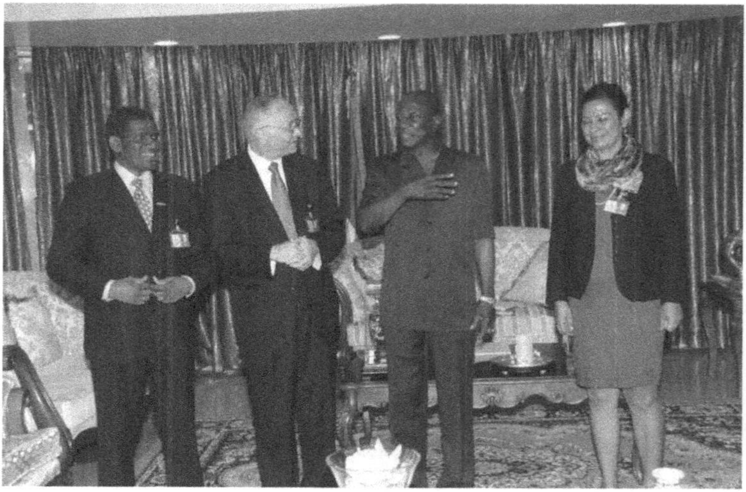

Dr. Sakoba, his wife and their children
The president with WHO executives

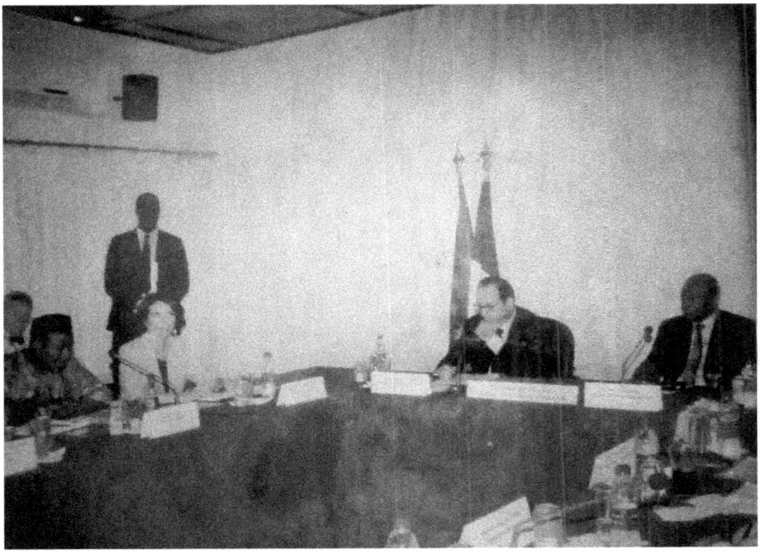

In company of President Francois Hollande

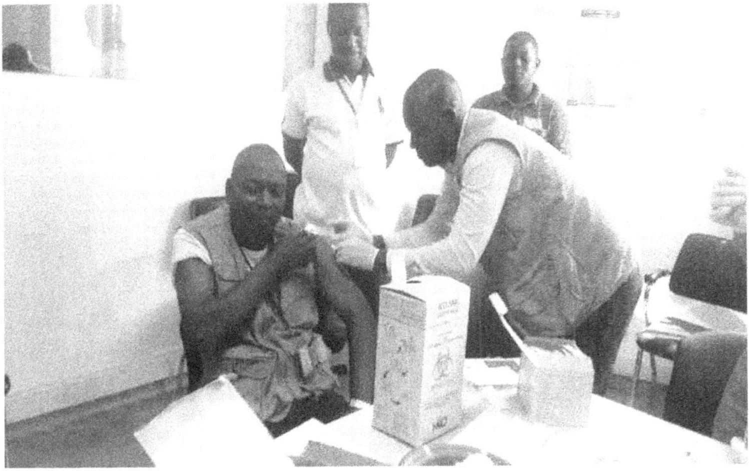

Launch of vaccination against Ebola (March 7th, 2015)

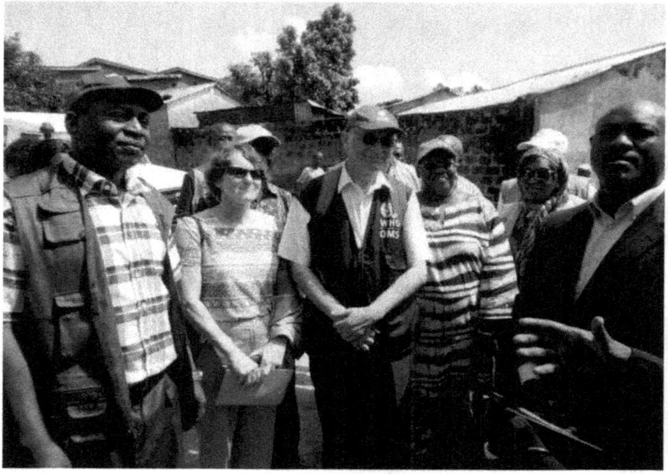

Field visit with the CDC country director, Lise Martel, and the WHO representative, Mohamed Belhocine

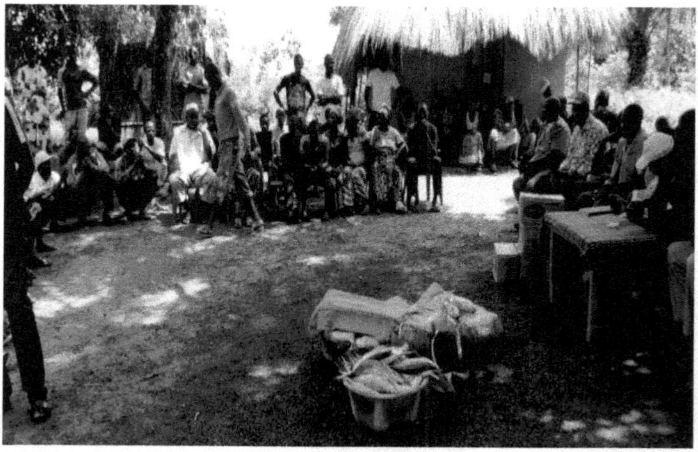

Sensitization session for the population of a village for the ring strapping (containment) of a positive case of Ebola

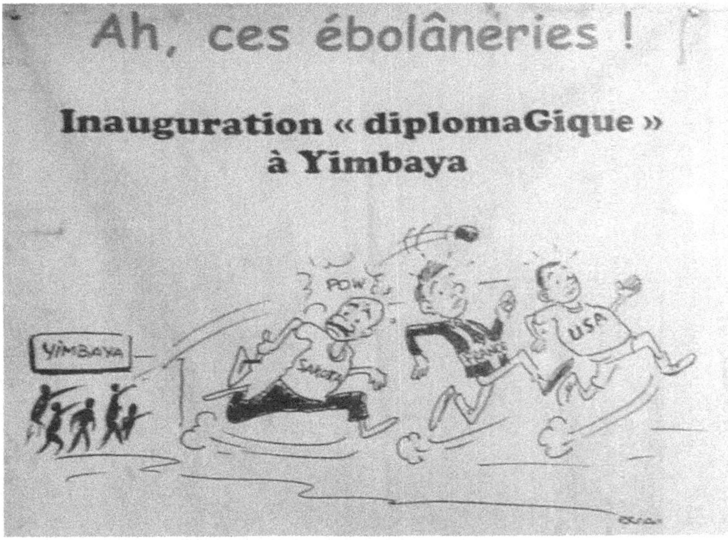

Caricature of a session

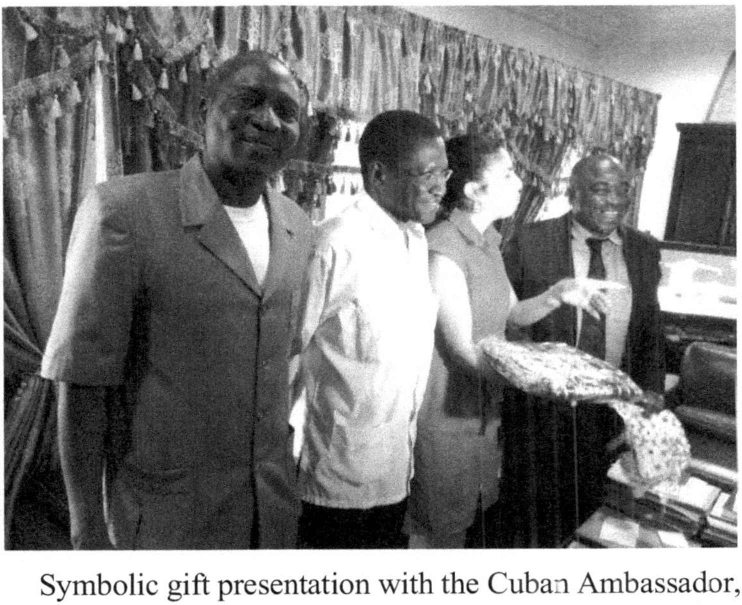

Symbolic gift presentation with the Cuban Ambassador, and the Minister of Health and his Secretary General

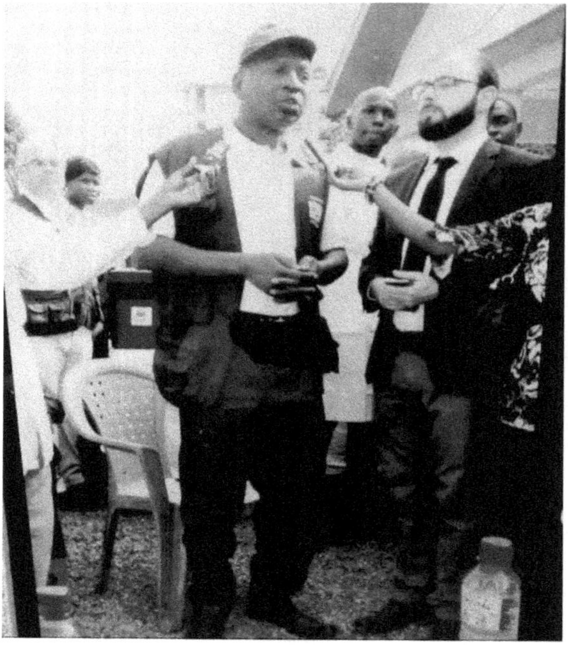

Presentation of the Legion of Honor by the French Ambassador

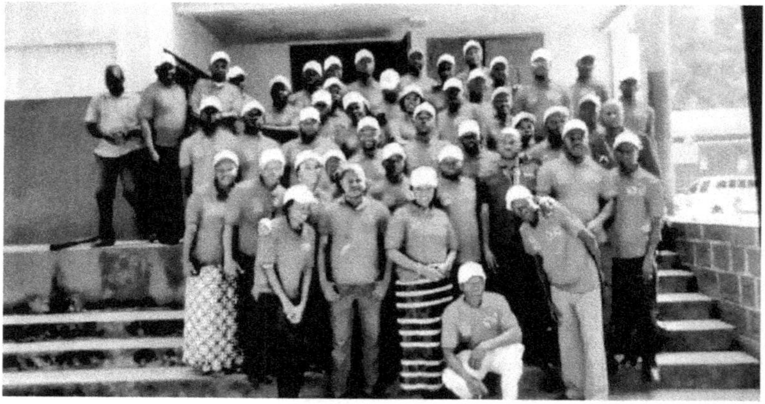

Interview with journalists during the vaccination launch

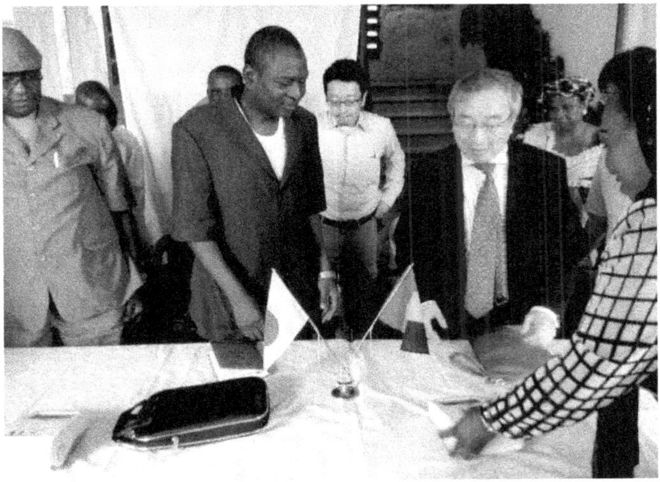

Training of the prefectoral alert and response teams (EPARE) for the fight against Ebola

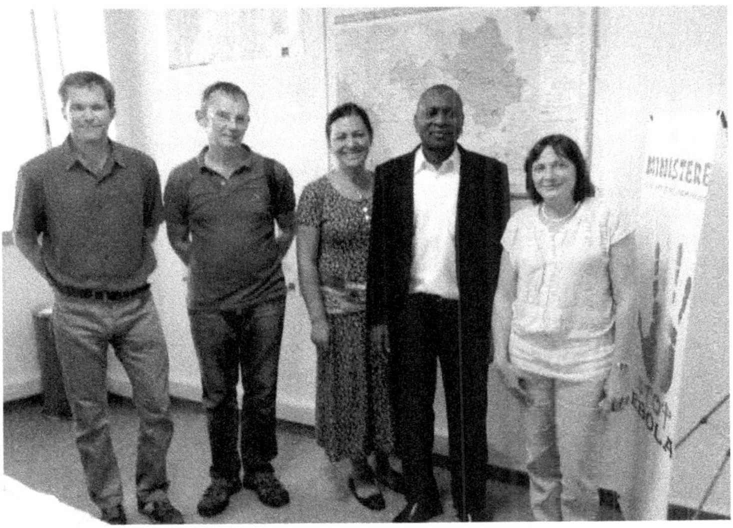

Ceremony of donation with the Japanese Ambassador

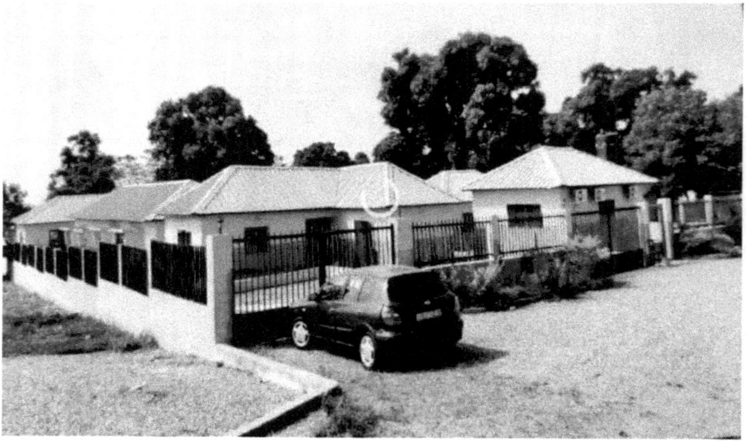

Preparation of the vaccination team led by Marie-Paule Kenny

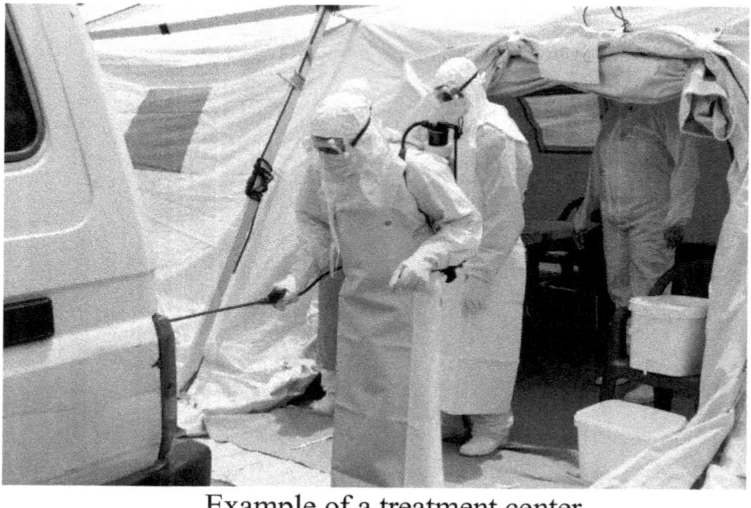

Example of a treatment center
Treatment team for Ebola

Table of contents

Structures éditoriales du groupe L'Harmattan

L'Harmattan Italie
Via degli Artisti, 15
10124 Torino
harmattan.italia@gmail.com

L'Harmattan Hongrie
Kossuth l. u. 14-16.
1053 Budapest
harmattan@harmattan hu

L'Harmattan Sénégal
10 VDN en face Mermoz
BP 45034 Dakar-Fann
senharmattan@gmail.com

L'Harmattan Cameroun
TSINGA/FECAFOOT
BP 11486 Yaoundé
inkoukam@gmail.com

L'Harmattan Burkina Faso
Achille Somé – tengnule@hotmail.fr

L'Harmattan Guinée
Almamya, rue KA 028 OKB Agency
BP 3470 Conakry
harmattanguinee@yahoo.fr

L'Harmattan RDC
185, avenue Nyangwe
Commune de Lingwala – Kinshasa
matangilamusadila@yahoo.fr

L'Harmattan Congo
67, boulevard Denis-Sassou-N'Guesso
BP 2874 Brazzaville
harmattan.congo@yahoo.fr

L'Harmattan Mali
Sirakoro-Meguetana V31
Bamako
syllaka@yahoo.fr

L'Harmattan Togo
Djidjole – Lomé
Maison Amela
face EPP BATOME
ddamela@aol.com

L'Harmattan Côte d'Ivoire
Résidence Karl – Cité des Arts
Abidjan-Cocody
03 BP 1588 Abidjan
espace_harmattan.ci@hotmail.fr

L'Harmattan Algérie
22, rue Moulay-Mohamed
31000 Oran
info2@harmattan-algerie.com

L'Harmattan Maroc
5, rue Ferrane-Kouicha, Talaâ-Elkbira
Chrableyine, Fès-Médine
30000 Fès
harmattan.maroc@gmail.com

Nos librairies en France

Librairie internationale
16, rue des Écoles – 75005 Paris
librairie.internationale@harmattan.fr
01 40 46 79 11
www.librairieharmattan.com

Librairie l'Espace Harmattan
21 bis, rue des Écoles – 75005 paris
librairie.espace@harmattan.fr
01 43 29 49 42

Lib. sciences humaines & histoire
21, rue des Écoles – 75005 paris
librairie.sh@harmattan.fr
01 46 34 13 71
www.librairieharmattansh.com

Lib. Méditerranée & Moyen-Orient
7, rue des Carmes – 75005 Paris
librairie.mediterranee@harmattan.fr
01 43 29 71 15

Librairie Le Lucernaire
53, rue Notre-Dame-des-Champs – 75006 Paris
librairie@lucernaire.fr
01 42 22 67 13

www.ingramcontent.com/pod-product-compliance
Lightning Source LLC
Chambersburg PA
CBHW071447230926
51846CB00001B/365
* 9 7 8 2 1 4 0 3 1 6 2 9 6 *